Managed Care in
Human Services

Managed Care in Human Services

Edited By
Stephen P. Wernet

LYCEUM
BOOKS, INC.

Chicago, Illinois

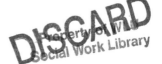

© Lyceum Books, Inc., 1999

Published by

LYCEUM BOOKS, INC.
5758 S. Blackstone Ave.
Chicago, Illinois 60637
773-643-1903 (Fax)
773-643-1902 (Phone)
lyceum3@:bm.net
http//www.lyceumbooks.com

Library of Congress Cataloging-in-Publication Data

Managed care in human services/edited by Stephen P. Wernet.
  p. cm.
  Includes bibliographical references and index.
  ISBN 0-925065-30-7 (alk. paper)
  1. Managed mental health care. 2. Child welfare--Effect of
managed care on. 3. Family services--Effect of managed care on. I.
Wernet, Stephen P., 1951-
  RC465.6 .M36 1999

ISBN 0-925065-30-7

Contents

CHAPTER 1

Introduction to Managed Care in Human Services

Stephen P. Wernet
Professor, School of Social Service
Saint Louis University

Although many social workers and human service professionals discuss it as if it were a recent phenomenon, managed care is nearly a decade old. Managed care has its conceptual and evolutionary roots in social movements and policies that date back to the early phases of the Great Society programs. In fact, managed care can be placed within a larger context of the competing values that have surrounded American social welfare policy since the advent of the nineteenth century. The purpose of this chapter is to provide the reader with an overview of managed care, its philosophy, its impact on service design and implementation and identify select issues of importance for managed care in human services.

THE ESSENCE OF MANAGED CARE

"Managed care" is a very elastic term used to describe a variety of health care financing methods and delivery systems. When people talk about managed care, they are referring to a system of delivering services and a system of care management (Broskowski, 1991; Corcoran & Vandiver, 1996; Hoge, Davidson, Griffith, Sledge, & Howenstine, 1994; Mechanic, Schlesinger, & McAlpine, 1995; Sederer & Bennett, 1996; Winegar, 1993). Managed care is an attempt to combine financial administration of a health care organization with responsible patient care.

Managed care has two overarching goals. They are to control costs while maintaining the quality of services. The objectives of managed health care is to design a system that enhances human values and sustains professional practice. It attempts to maximize both the use of advances in knowledge and technology and the economies of scale associated with large-scale organizations. It is both cost containment and clinical decision making.

The problem is that these two goals are usually competing and, according to some people, mutually exclusive. On the one hand, there is the drive to provide accessible, comprehensive, continuous, and effective services, which, on the other hand, is tempered by the recognition that resources are scarce and cost efficiency needed. As some people describe it, managed health care pits cost against quality (Sederer & Bennett, 1996; Sederer & St. Clair, 1990; Webb, 1987).

Cost Containment versus High Quality

Managed care began with private industry's wish to contain health care expenditures (Broskowski, 1991; Finkelstein & Frissel, 1990; Root, 1991). In particular, it began with a focus on physical health care and its costs. As the cost of health care increased, private industry sought ways to limit and even reduce these costs. Three approaches to health care cost containment emerged. The first solution involved decreasing the extent of health care coverage provided by employers for employees. This solution was adopted as a means of maintaining health care costs at their current levels of expenditure. The second solution involved decreasing the amount paid by employers for health care while increasing copayment costs for employees. This solution was adopted as a means of shifting health care costs to the consumer. It was often used when the consumer wanted more health care options, either services or providers, than the employer was willing or able to absorb into its budget.

These first two solutions of decreased coverage and increased cost shifting were attempts to contain the cost of health care for the employer. They were consumer-focused solutions. In both solutions, the emphasis was on limiting the choices and costs of the consumer, and the provider or expense side of the health care system was ignored.

However, these solutions were unsuccessful in containing the health care costs for industry (Browkowski, 1991; DeLeon, VandenBos, & Bulatao, 1991; Webber, 1995), and so another solution was attempted. This third solution is known as managed care. It involves improving the match between the service needed or desired by the consumer and the service provided by the health care professional or system. It is related to the earlier system of diagnosis-related groups. These treatment groupings associated the rate of reimbursement with a previously determined, and appropriate, course of treatment for the diagnosed illness or injury. Managed care focuses on both sides of the health care equation: consumer and provider.

The managed care solution has several goals. The first is constraint of the autonomous decision making of the medical practitioner. This is an attempt to standardize solutions to health problems thereby enabling comparability of treatment and costs. The second goal is use of generic treatment. This is an attempt to eliminate particularistic treatment thereby reducing costs for equally effective regimens. The third goal is redesign of the health care sys-

tem away from institution based care and delivery of health care services—
that is, hospital-based delivery of care—and toward community-based care
and delivery of health care services. This is an attempt to exploit newer treatment technology and knowledge thereby, again, reducing costs for equally
effective treatment.

As a solution for physical health care, managed care, and its older rela-
tives, has started to have some impact on health care costs. For example,
insurers and employers are less amenable to open-ended health care services
and unrestrained use of health care procedures (Dorwart & Schlesinger, 1988;
Levin, Glasser, & Jaffee, 1988). The result of this new health care management
approach has been fewer inpatient procedures and briefer inpatient stays (Fre-
und & Hurley, 1995; Sederer & Bennett, 1996). These results have led to
lower patient census and lower bed occupancy (Christianson et al., 1995;
Reed, Hennessy, Mitchell, & Babigian, 1994). Consequently, hospitals are not
recovering the full amount of their expenses (Belkin, 1996).

An outgrowth of these initiatives has been the merger, acquisition, and
joint venture frenzy occurring among health care institutions today. Similar
institutions combine and recombine into larger and larger health care systems
with fewer options for consumers. The argument that has been offered is that
in order to achieve the economies of scale that will make delivery of services
affordable, large interlocking networks of health care providers must be created from among the small, independent health care providers. This new
health care supersystem is beginning to come precariously close to a monop-
oly.

These approaches to cost containment have been successful with physical health care. However, there is another side to the health care equation.
This other side is behavioral health care and incorporates the arenas of substance abuse and mental health services.

The historical outcome of cost containment in behavioral health care
has been, at best, mixed. It has been notoriously expensive to consume and
deliver behavioral health care service. Certainly, less is known about what type
of service works effectively with which clinical problem constellation, and
therefore, about how much time is necessary for treatment to remedy a given
behavioral health problem.

This uncertainty has led to several different approaches to behavioral
health care (Christianson & Gray, 1994; Fennell & Alexander, 1993; Frank,
McGuire, & Newhouse, 1995; Schinnar, Rothbard, & Hadley, 1992). One
approach is to integrate behavioral health care into the physical health care
system or service so that it is subject to the same review and cost containment
procedure and process. This is referred to as an *integrated system*. Behavioral
health care services are part and parcel of a system in which the provider must
cover all aspects of health care.

Another approach is to partially integrate behavioral health care into the
physical health care system. This approach is referred to as a *carved-in system*.

Behavioral health care is part of a health care system, but usually there are pre-determined limits on the amount or type of services provided by the health care system.

And yet another approach is to exempt or exclude behavioral health care from the physical health care system. This approach removes behavioral health care from the sets of health care procedures and processes while subjecting it to a uniquely designed and specifically defined set of review and cost containment procedures and processes. Behavioral health care is provided independent of physical health care. This last approach is referred to as a *carved-out system*. It is euphemistically referred to as behavioral health care carve-out.

The early example of behavioral health care in a managed system is found in employee assistance programs (EAPs; Finkelstein & Frissel, 1990; Mullady, 1991; Root, 1991). These programs were, and continue to be, integral components in human resource departments and benefit packages. They are typically part of and integrated with the brief, or emergency, medical care facilities on the business campus. Some work sites, such as General Motors assembly plants, have very large medical care facilities; others, such as a white-collar office, have virtually nothing on site. Some companies offer in-house EAP services; others purchase or outsource the services to a contractor or agent. Some services are remedial only; some services are a broad-brush approach that also offers preventive and educational programs. All three contemporary approaches to behavioral health care are exemplified through employee assistance.

Managed care arose to address rising costs in physical health care. The solutions tended to develop in serial response. When focused on the consumer, managed care sought to constrict choice in treatment resource or to shift expenses to contain costs. When focused on the provider, managed care sought to constrict treatment choices through standardization and use of generic solutions, or to shift venue for delivery of treatment. In the behavioral health care arena, however, solutions have been integrated and parallel, addressing consumer and provider simultaneously. These solutions have yielded the complex, interconnected system to which we now turn our attention.

The Essence of a Managed Care System

Every managed care system has three levels (see table 1). These are the policy-making level, the system design level, and the service provider level. The policy-making level of the managed care system is concerned with the grand perspective or overview of the system. It focuses on setting general policy that will guide the managed care system. This primary level is concerned with a broad outline of how to achieve both cost containment and high-quality services. This dual goal is usually accomplished by attempting to balance benefit offerings, number of visits, annual cost outlay, lifetime expenditure, deductibles, and copayments.

Table 1   Structure of a Managed Care System

Level	Focus
1. Policy making	Establishes general policy guidelines for achieving cost containment and high-quality services
2. System design and implementation	Design service system Establish treatment protocols Implement gatekeeping operations Implement utilization review and quality assurance mechanisms
3. Service provider network	Select and certify/qualify provider for network

In the private sector, the policy-making level addresses such issues as the type of health care provided to the employees of the company. It will also establish a stance on whether the organization will deliver services directly, manage the benefit system, or buy the assorted services, management and direct, from an outside vendor. This is sometimes referred to as the decision to "make" (deliver services by the policy-making body) or "buy" (purchase services from an outside vendor).

In the public sector, policy making addresses the scope of the state or code agencies' responsibilities and the target population(s) for service. At this level, decisions will be made about the level of state agencies' participation in delivery of services and about which populations and services will be served through carved-out approaches. The decision to carve out services and populations usually focuses on the consumers with highest need—the most vulnerable, the most needy, and the severely chronic individuals within the care of the state agency. Chapter 2 describes how the carve-out decision plays out in child welfare systems, while chapters 4 and 9 depict these issues as they occur in mental health systems. The policy-making level is concerned with the broad eligibility criteria for inclusion in the system. Decisions may also focus on consolidating several different funding streams. For example, chapter 4 discusses the use of Medicaid funds to support a single-payer and single-provider system in Massachusetts. The Calgary Rockyview community, described in chapter 5, consolidates funds into one envelope for use in supporting a redesigned, consolidated, and comprehensive child and family service system.

The second level of the managed care system is system design and implementation. This level focuses on configuration of the delivery system and the choice of implementing agent. This second level is executed through a combination of policy-making body and administrative service organization, that is, the purchasing agent of the outside vendor.

There are four different elements at the system design level of managed care. The first element is the design of the service system itself. The design typically outlines the range of services that will be purchased for and on behalf of the consumer. Terms such as "continuum of care" or an "array of services" are used when this aspect of the second level is discussed. This is where the "make or buy" decision of the policy-making level is implemented.

The second element is establishment of treatment protocols. Decision criteria are established for linking consumer problem with appropriate treatment. This approach assumes that for every presenting problem there is a best practice to addressing it.

The third element is the gatekeeping function. This function is responsible for approving delivery and ultimately payment for services delivered by an approved or willing provider. It is the initial point of contact, through which the consumer for whom services are purchased must pass in order to receive services from an approved service provider.

The fourth element is the review mechanism. This mechanism is usually referred to as utilization review and quality assurance. It has two goals: 1) to ensure that service providers are following the proper course of treatment and 2) to review treatment protocols for effectiveness.

The third level of a managed care system is the network of service providers that are used in it. This network may take any number of different forms or structures. The general principle is certifying or qualifying a provider who is willing to or interested in serving as a resource for the consumer to be served. The term typical is "any willing, qualified provider" (Keigher, 1995; Sederer & St. Clair, 1990). This phase has two important components. The first is *qualified*. This term refers to a professional service provider, typically an individual, who has been investigated and found worthwhile for inclusion in the service provider network. This investigation focuses on the credentials and preparation of the potential provider. The goal of the investigation or certification is to select the best trained individuals for the service network. An additional purpose is to identify and select into the network providers with unique or unusual skills that are presently unavailable within the network service array or continuum of services.

The second concept in the phrase is *willing*. This term refers to a provider's agreement to work within the guidelines and constraints of the system. This agreement includes client referrals, treatment protocols, and reimbursement rates.

Every managed care system has three levels: a policy-making level, a system design and implementation level, and a service provider network level. These levels may be consolidated within one organization (for example, state child welfare agency or mental health department), or they may be dissociated from each other in order to function as checks and balances (for example, purchased or contracted social services and service auditing for nonprofit and proprietary organizations in conjunction with state agency policy setting).

Chapter 6 and 7 provide different examples of system design. Chapter 6 depicts the coexistence of implementation and provider levels within one organization. Divisional structures were instituted to separate the two levels thereby ensuring integrity of the system. Chapter 7 depicts the traditional approach of separate organizational homes as the means of separating the system's levels of operation. It is to system implementation that we now turn our attention.

The Essence of Managed Care Implementation

When implemented, a managed care system has five essential elements (see table 2). These include capitation and performance contracting, deflection from substitute care, preauthorization, utilization review, and case management of higher-volume users. These elements aim to contain costs while ensuring high-quality services. They cut across the system design and service provider levels.

The first essential element of a managed care system is *capitation and performance contracting* (Broskowski, 1991; Christianson & Gray, 1994; Cole, Reed, Babigian, Brown, & Fray, 1994; Frank et al., 1995; Freeborn & Pope, 1994; Grimaldi, 1996; Schinnar et al., 1989). Capitation is a payment system through which a provider receives a set, predetermined dollar amount per participant or potential participant in a catchment area or targeted population of the managed care system. Capitation is based on a formula that pays a certain rate of dollars per person regardless of the individual's utilization of services. The formula is constructed from four data elements: historical data on service use, historical data on costs for services, actuarial projections of potential use, and actuarial projection of potential costs for services. The formula employs a smoothing philosophy for spreading costs and risks across the entire target population. Assuming continuity of trends, capitation relies on comprehensive and detailed data of historical use as well as statistical modeling of future demand. Therefore, capitation requires sophisticated management information systems tracking both cost and service history.

Although capitation formulas have been used in physical health care, they have been less routinely applied in human services. The use of Medicaid funding and hospital providers has given mental health services some experience with capitation, as discussed in both chapters 4 and 9. By contrast, however, the dearth of data and data system problems in child welfare, described in chapters 2 and 3, make the use of capitation formulas problematic in this arena. Contracting for child welfare services under managed care is consequently challenging at best.

Another aspect of this first essential element is performance contracting. Performance contracting is an approach that is becoming increasingly popular in the public sector. It is a management approach that melds purchase-of-service contracting with capitation. Purchase-of-service contracting reim-

Table 2   Elements of a Managed Care System

Element	Concepts
1. Capitation and performance contracting	Capitation: formula-based payment for services to be rendered Performance contracting: reimbursement based on impact of provided services
2. Deflection from substitute care	Substitutability Comparability of services Treatment in least restrictive environment Cost efficiency
3. Preauthorization	Gatekeeping
4. Utilization review	Efficiency of treatment Treatment protocols
5. Case management of high-volume users	

burses providers for services based on units of service delivered. Performance contracting divides the reimbursement process into a tripartite payment system. It combines a start-up cost block payment, partial reimbursement for actual units of services delivered, and a final payment for services rendered based on demonstration of successful treatment after a predetermined time period following termination of service. An example of performance contracting is job training for recipients of temporary aid to needy families (TANF). Agencies or businesses that provide job training to TANF recipients receive a proportion of the contract as start-up costs, receive another proportion of the total contract over its life as services are provided, and receive a final payment for the balance of the contract either three or six months after the training period provided the trainee is still employed. Although there is no set formula for performance contract payment systems, it is typical to see 25% start-up payment, and 50% reimbursement over the life of the contract, and a final 25% payment if the performance target is reached successfully at the specified date.

Capitation and performance contracting have a common philosophy. This philosophy is known as *risk assumption*. In both contractual arrangements, the provider assumes a certain amount of financial risk for the services provided. Under capitation, if services that are rendered cost more than the capitated payment rate, the provider absorbs those costs. Under performance contracting, if the performance target is not achieved, the final payment on the contract is not made to the provider. These approaches to risk sharing are thought to curtail costs because the provider has a vested interest in the success of the system. If the services are unsuccessful, the provider is liable for expenses. Therefore, it behooves the provider to treat judiciously under capitation and accurately under performance contracting. In both cases, the provider absorbs the costs of treatment mistakes.

The second essential element in an implemented managed care system is *deflection from substitute care* (Abbott, Jordan, & Murtaza, 1995; Dorwart & Schlesinger, 1988; Mechanic et al., 1995). Deflection from substitute care is the operationalization of the concept of substitutability. Substitutability is built on three different ideas: comparability of services, least restrictive environment, and cost efficiency. The first idea is use of *comparable treatment services*. It suggests there are certain services that can be used in lieu of other services. The substituted services will produce outcomes as good as the original constellation but at lower cost. This philosophy operates in child welfare through the use of family preservation and wraparound services in lieu of either foster care or residential placement of children. A constellation of services can be used with a family as a substitute for foster care or out-of-home placement. This philosophy is also evident in mental health services where a combination of services is used as a substitute for hospitalizing the severely and profoundly mentally ill. A constellation of services such as medication monitoring, supervised group home living, and sheltered workshops are used in lieu of institutionalization. Chapters 2 and 3 discuss this idea as applied in child welfare. Chapters 8 and 9 describe cases in which substitutability has been attempted for both child welfare and mental health services.

The second idea that undergirds deflection from substitute care is use of *least restrictive environment*. Least restrictive environment is both a treatment and a legal idea that has evolved in human services in the past thirty to forty years. It is a philosophy that is grounded in the movement to protect the civil rights of the mentally ill and to promote deinstitutionalization. The philosophy of least restrictive environment espouses the idea that wherever and whenever possible, the client or recipient of services should be assisted in an environment that most closely resembles a normal living environment, maximizes the individual's personal choices, and protects the individual's freedom. This philosophy was borne from numerous class action suits brought on behalf of the mentally ill in numerous state institutions throughout the country. Over time, evidence has emerged that service outcomes are as good in a less restrictive environment as in a more restrictive one (Feild, 1996; Tuma, 1989). For example, the use of group homes for the mentally ill when combined with shelter workshops are as good in preparing individuals to live in a community as treatment services in state institutions (Behar, 1985, 1990; Levendusky, Willis, & Ghinassi, 1994).

The third idea within substitutability is the idea of *cost efficiency*. This idea has evolved from comparability of treatment services and least restrictive environment philosophies. Cost efficiency and substitutability imply that if one is able to obtain the same outcome at a lower cost, then one should use, or substitute, the less costly treatment. In physical health care, this idea has resulted in reduction of patients' postsurgical lengths of stay in hospitals. It has also resulted in the use of outpatient surgical procedures in lieu of inpatient surgeries. In human services, this idea has been evidenced by the use of family preservation services in lieu of placement for at-risk and neglected children. In mental health, it has been evidenced by the use of supervised community living, supervised work, and medication monitoring in lieu of hospitalization of the severely and profoundly mentally ill individual.

The consequences can be bad or good. Chapter 4 reports on one pitfall of substitutability for cost efficiency through overreliance on medication in lieu of therapeutic services. Chapters 8 and 9, however, report on valuable innovations in alternative service approaches to achieve cost efficiencies within human systems. For example, intensive crisis intervention and introduction of an array of services have proved effective at preventing the need for some hospitalizations and child placements.

The third essential element of a managed care system is *preauthorization* (Broskowski, 1991; Hoge et al., 1994; Winegar, 1993). This component is sometimes referred to as precertification or gatekeeping. Preauthorization serves two major purposes. First, preauthorization attempts to match the need of the client with the appropriate service within the system. Its goal is to ensure receipt of the appropriate service given the presenting problem or difficulty of the individual. The second goal or preauthorization is cost containment. Cost containment has several aspects. The first is to limit access to costly services. This aspect of preauthorization reflects managed care's concerns with capitation and risk management. By constraining consumers' use of costly services, a managed care system attempts to constrain cost of services.

Limiting access works in conjunction with the second aspect of preauthorization—substitutability. It is assumed that a substituted service is less costly and, therefore, cheaper for the system. By finding an appropriate, suitable, equivalent alternative approach to service that can be substituted for the most costly service and still achieve appropriate if not identical outcomes, a managed care system is reducing costs. By substituting less costly services, the system is able to limit overall expenses for the service package to the managed care system and ultimately the consumer who pays the bill.

In the process of matching client need to appropriate service, and using substitutability, the managed care system is addressing a third aspect. It is attempting to apply and balance two different decision criteria. These criteria are *medical necessity* and *clinical appropriateness*. Through medical necessity, a managed care system and its gatekeeper(s) are attempting to match client need with available service(s). Medical necessity maintains that there is a variety of treatments that can be used to satisfy the clients' need for service. Any one of these treatments may be as good as another and, therefore, the least expensive service can be implemented to meet the client's needs. On the other hand, clinical appropriateness emphasizes the best treatment services for the client irrespective of the cost of the service. Clinical appropriateness argues for the single best treatment for the client even though there may be several different treatments that can be employed to meet the client's service needs. Where medical necessity argues for a generic treatment protocol and use of the least expensive treatment modality, clinical appropriateness argues for an individualized and unique treatment package.

Chapters 6, 9, and 10 report on the tensions that exist among clinicians with regard to these criteria. Many clinicians are inclined to see clinical appropriateness and a client's individuality and uniqueness as synonymous. They tend to use open-ended treatment because they have an antimeasurement bias. These attitudes are changing slowly as brief treatment becomes more widely accepted and as more clinicians are trained in it. Clinicians are beginning to realize that brief treatment is not antithetical to a client's individuality. This change may help speed efforts to measure therapeutic change thereby enhancing our understanding of medical necessity in the human services.

The fourth element of a managed care system is *utilization review* (Allen, 1993; Hoge et al., 1994; Mechanic et al., 1995; Sederer & St. Clair, 1990). It is the process by which treatment effectiveness and service outcome is assessed by the managed care system. It is concerned with the efficacy of treatment and treatment protocol.

There are two approaches to utilization review. They can be used either independent of each other or simultaneously. These approaches are *concurrent* utilization review and *retrospective* utilization review. Concurrent utilization review takes place during the treatment process. Its goal is to evaluate the effectiveness of the service treatment protocol as it is presently being implemented. Retrospective utilization review is concerned with reviewing the efficacy and implementation of service treatment protocols after a service has been delivered and a case closed. In both cases, utilization review addresses several issues. First is the implementation of treatment protocol. Here, utilization review is concerned with whether the treatment services that have been outlined as necessary and appropriate for a particular problem were implemented. The second issue is impact assessment. Here utilization review is concerned with the efficacy of treatment. Was treatment as delivered for the client's problem effective in remediating the client's problem? If the treatment was successful, then utilization review is complete. If, on the other hand, treatment was unsuccessful or worked better than anticipated, utilization review moves to a third issue—review and revision of the treatment protocol. If the treatment was unsuccessful, utilization review seeks to learn why. If treatment was better than anticipated, utilization review also wants to learn why. Utilization review depends on accurate and timely data collection at the point of clinical service in the system. It depends on valid and reliable measurement of both client's problem and treatment intervention.

Measurement of both intervention and outcome is difficult, and human service professionals tend to resist the measurement process. Performance measurement needs to focus on three areas: treatment process, treatment outcome, and client satisfaction (Martin & Kettner, 1996). Unfortunately, managed care systems and subcontracted providers have come to rely on indirect, tertiary measures of impact in lieu of well-designed outcome assessments systems. These measures include provider credentialing and client satisfaction. With provider credentialing, a managed care system focuses on the level of education, type of training, and professional experience of the service provider. It is believed that the use of credentialing ensures that high-quality services are being delivered. By extension, it is believed that established treatment protocols are being appropriately implemented.

The second measure that is substituted for well-designed impact assessment is client satisfaction surveys. These surveys are typically collected at two points in time. The first is at termination of service delivery, the second at some time in the future. The future date varies, depending on the system, anywhere from one month to one year after termination of services. Once again, client satisfaction surveys rely on the assumption of an indirect effect. That is, if the client is satisfied then the treatment must be successful. Unfortunately,, these types of assessment systems are highly susceptible to social acquiescence. Chapter 4, for example, highlights some of the difficulties with satisfaction measures as a surrogate for outcome and impact assessments. Utilization review is one of the greatest challenges for managed care in the human services.

The fifth element of a managed care system is *case management* of high-volume users (Goldstein, Bassuk, Holland, & Zimmer, 1988; Sederer & Bennett, 1996). This element is one of the newer components of managed care systems and may not be present in all systems. This feature, however, appears to be present in most public sector managed care systems. Case management is an attempt to monitor the use and impact of services for a select group of users who need multiple and numerous services. The "high-volume user" is defined by each system, but in general, this term refers to a user who demonstrates an extraordinarily high level of service consumption, which places him or her outside a usual, customary, and normal range of variance for amount of services used as defined by the treatment protocol in a managed care system. In both operation and philosophy, case management of high-volume users resembles utilization review. Unlike utilization review, however, case management of high-volume users seeks to move the user out of the treatment system through the combination of various services rather than testing for the efficacy of the services. Little is known about the efficacy of case management of high-volume users. It is probable that this feature will become a standard aspect of managed care systems.

In summary, a managed care system will have five elements that address cost and utilization. Capitation and performance contracting are formulaic approaches to spreading costs and risks based on historical trends and actual performance. Deflection from substitute care espouses alternative treatment approaches as a way to contain costs and service utilization. Preauthorization focuses on matching clients' needs with suitable services as a means of controlling service utilization. Utilization review is concerned with assessing treatment effectiveness in order to control costs and service constellations. Case management of high-volume users attempts to ensure appropriate service utilization as a means of controlling costs.

SELECT ISSUES CONCERNING MANAGED CARE IN HUMAN SERVICES

Select issues within managed care have potential impact on human services. These include cost shifting, continuity of care, community-based care and the role of the community, gatekeeping and decision-making criteria, and accountability.

Cost Shifting

One of the hidden goals of managed care is to shift the cost of services away from the historical, principal purchaser of services to both the direct consumer of service and the provider of service. Cost shifting is intended to reallocate the risk associated with service expenditures and thereby contain the costs associated with services.

Risk reallocation as a component of cost containment has been attributed directly to the exponential growth in health care costs (Belkin, 1996; Broskowski, 1991; Frank et al., 1995; Freeborn & Pope, 1995; McGuire, 1994). Cost shifting reflects a dramatic philosophical change in the concept of health care benefits. No longer a fringe benefit of the employee provided by the employer—that is, a public good—it is treated as an individual responsibility subject to marketplace consumerism, introducing a private goods approach to health care. The employer has backed away from responsibility for health care while retaining some share of the cost and shifting some to the employee.

The unique aspect of cost shifting under managed care is that the provider of service is asked to assume risk associated with the cost of delivering services under contract. Employers and employees have turned to providers and are demanding that they take some responsibility for cost overruns and cost containment. Providers who accept some of the burden will be incorporated into the service provider network. Those who do not will be excluded.

The typical approach to cost sharing is fixed cost reimbursement. The fixed cost reimbursement contract has been used for several decades by health maintenance organizations such as Kaiser Permanente. In recent years, however, risk assumption in the form of cost shifting has become a standard operating practice in health care and human services.

Cost shifting has also been present in public human services for several decades. It can take the form of less than full reimbursement under purchase-of-service contracting between state agencies and human service providers. Or it can take the form of match requirements under such programs as Title XX. However, unlike cost sharing and less than full reimbursement, cost shifting and risk assumption make no provision for deficit financing in the event of cost overruns. Cost shifting, therefore, requires pinpoint accuracy in projection of cost, revenue, and service consumption. These types of projections require sophisticated information management, which has been largely underdeveloped in human services.

Another aspect of cost shifting is consolidation of funding streams. This has become prevalent as a response to the devoution of federal participation in social welfare programming for vulnerable populations. As the federal government has reduced its contribution to and funding of social welfare programming, state, county, and local governments have become creative and innovative at accessing existing systems of federal revenue not previously used for vulnerable populations. This approach has enabled nonfederal entities to retain programming for vulnerable populations at or near current levels while maintaining their current level of support, and not raising taxes. Part of the success of this strategy has been attributed to the flush economy (Feild, 1996; Salamon, 1993). An example of this approach is the use of Medicaid funds to underwrite the costs of community-based mental health programs for the severely and profoundly mentally ill. Community-based agencies become accredited as Medicaid certified organizations or rehabilitation certified organizations, thereby becoming eligible for Medicaid reimbursement for services provided to the severely and profoundly mentally ill.

However, as they confront continuing reduction of federal health and human services dollars, states are pursuing their own approaches to funding stream consolidation. States are seeking and receiving waivers to merge various funding streams, such as Medicaid and Medicare with mental health and social service funds, into single-fund pools to purchase physical and behavioral health services for vulnerable populations. With these consolidations, the states are looking to maximize not only the efficiency of delivered services but also the number of services available for set amounts of dollars. Service providers are contracted to deliver a full array of services for set reimbursement. General expectations for assumption of cost overruns by the providers are incorporated into the negotiated contracts. This outlines the risk that will be assumed by all parties, especially the provider, thereby shifting new responsibilities to the providers and the service networks.

Several contributors to this volume discuss these consolidations. Chapter 4 reports on cost shifting to Medicaid in order to meet mental health needs in the Commonwealth of Massachusetts. Chapter 5 reports on a Canadian effort to develop a single, consolidated funding stream for child and family services. Chapters 6 through 9 describe the impact of consolidated funding on provider organizations. As revenue is reduced and consolidated by administrative service organizations, providers must find new revenue sources or developing structures that ensure organizational survival.

Continuity of Care

The second select issue is continuity of care. This idea is known by a number of different names—for example, comprehensive services, continuum of care, and array of services (Bickman, 1996; Golant & McCaslin, 1979; Hicks & Bopp, 1996; Levendusky et al., 1994; Morrison Dore, Wilkerson, & Sonis, 1992; Shortell et al., 1996; Watkins & Watkins, 1984). The concept refers to two related elements: seamlessness of services and availability of services. *Seamlessness* describes the ability of consumers to move between services without a break in continuity of treatment. It means that a client can move between intensity of services, usually from more intense to less intense, without either delay or disruption of preexisting therapeutic relationships. In physical health care, seamlessness is usually addressed through the use of a primary care physician. This individual knows the consumer and serves as the link between various specialists. In behavioral health care, seamlessness is typically addressed through the use of a case manager. This individual serves as the coordinator of services for the consumer. In behavioral health, however, seamlessness has an additional connotation. It also refers to the ability of a consumer to retain a therapeutic relationship while moving to another level of service intensity. By retaining this meaningful relationship, it is believed that the consumer will maintain the gains achieved and not lose ground while moving into new relationships.

The second element, *availability of services,* is usually mentioned in the context of a continuum of care or an array of services. These terms refer to a range of service options available for use by consumers and treating agents. Regardless of the type of human service, including physical health care, the range of services extends from total care, such as twenty-four-hour substitute care in child welfare residential treatment facilities or psychiatric hospitalization, to supportive work, such as the mutual aid of Alcoholics Anonymous and Saint Vincent DePaul Societies. The philosophy is that a service provider should match the client's level of functioning with services that complement strengths and supplement weaknesses so that it is the consumer's needs, and not the provider's ability, that determine treatment. The assumption that undergirds this concept is that one can match a service with a need at every conceivable point along the continuum and in the array.

Community-Based Care and the Role of the Community

The third select issue is community-based care and the role of the community. Community-based care is both a philosophy and an approach to human services. As a philosophy, it maintains that the best places to treat a person are those that most closely resemble the person's natural environment. Community-based care evolves from the concept of normalization (Morrissey & Goldman, 1986). It mirrors the concept of least restrictive environment, in which clients have the right to treatment in places with the greatest personal freedom and least personal constraints (Bickman, 1996; Morrison Dore et al., 1992; Morrissey & Goldman, 1986).

As an approach, community-based care leads to development of and dependence on a continuum of care. On the one hand, this continuum results in deflection of consumers from substitute care facilities. On the other hand, it results in the development of intensive, twenty-four-hour treatment services in the community. In child welfare, the result is development of family preservation services and family foster care; in mental health, supervised group living and supported work environments; in juvenile corrections, intensive tracking services. These approaches are bolstered by cost-benefit analyses of human services, which have generally failed to demonstrate the efficacy of substitute care for enhancing child well-being, family functioning, and independent living (Behar, 1985, 1990; Feild, 1996; Mordock, 1996).

Community-based care has stimulated a new understanding of and role for the community. Under managed care in human services, the community, as the natural environment of the client, becomes the locus of treatment activity. As the locus of treatment, the community should be involved in the assessment and governance of the array of services. In some areas, this concept is known as a local area network (LAN). In other areas, it is called a comprehensive community network structure (CCNS). The role of community in the LAN is more circumscribed than in the CCNS. Within a LAN, the community is defined as constituted by the provider organizations. Within a CCNS, the community encompasses the provider organizations and the general citizenry who may or may not have existing ties with the provider organizations but have some interest in the array of services. (Chapter 5 reports on the development of one such CCNS.) This broader conception is sometimes referred to as a community of interest (Hunter & Riger, 1986), as opposed to a geographically bounded community (Rothman, 1996). The later is tied together simply by places of residence, which in today's world is a weak link for community. The former is linked by a shared interest in the well-being of others that transcends geographical boundaries. In the best of all worlds, communities of interest intersect with communities of place, resulting in rich and enmeshed natural networks.

Gatekeeping and Decision-Making Criteria

The fourth select issue is gatekeeping and decision-making criteria. Gatekeeping entails three tasks: ensuring that a defined target population receives appropriate services, limiting access to costly services, and diverting consumers to less intensive treatment modalities. Gatekeeping is intended to achieve several goals. These goals are matching consumer service needs to appropriate services and capping costs for services. The matching system is thought necessary because providers often appear to use the services that are most familiar, most comfortable, and most beneficial *to them*. The services so chosen are rarely the less costly ones. Cost-effectiveness studies, however, find no greater impact of more, or most, costly over less costly services.

Gatekeeping operationalizes a belief that if consumers' needs are met by appropriate services, costs will be lower for all parties in the managed care system. It uses substitutability of services to contain costs to patient, purchaser, and provider.

The barrier that gatekeeping must hurdle is decision-making criteria. How does one efficiently match need with service, and yet account for individuality of response or variance in treatment impact? Managed care's answer is to establish criteria that will be used to elect treatment protocols and judge the quality of care that is delivered to consumers (Nyberg & Marschke, 1993; Spath, 1993). The choice of criteria is informed by treatment philosophy, treatment focus, and systems control. Ultimately, however, it often reduces to a bald choice between two extremes: medical necessity or clinical appropriateness.

The criterion of *medical necessity* emphasizes acute care, prevention, short-term treatment, and generic treatment protocols. It assumes that there is a generic approach to treating a medical or behavioral condition. When applied correctly, this generic approach will be successful. However, medical necessity does not take into account the individual's response to the treatment protocol. In physical health care, this omission is reflected in the refusal to use stronger, and more expensive, medications when more common forms of therapeutics are ineffective or, worse yet, when the consumer is allergic to the medication. In behavioral health care, medical necessity manifests itself in the blanket application of one service, such as short-term outpatient counseling, when some clients require more intense services, such as choremakers or foster care.

Clinical appropriateness focuses on chronic care, prevention of remission, long-term treatment, and individualized treatment protocols. It assumes that every client has unique service needs that cannot be satisfied by a generic treatment protocol. In theory, this is true. However, clinical appropriateness does not acknowledge that most consumers can respond favorably to a generic treatment protocol.

When managed health care was initially conceived, it was intended to meld low cost with high-quality care. The goal was to develop the most cost effective, broadest array of services with the least amount of practice variation. Hence the push for treatment protocols. Managed care has succeeded in implementing the gatekeeper function and maximizing economic efficiency and in limiting use of the most sophisticated, most expensive technologies. It has been less successful in demonstrating that treatment protocols are flexible enough to allow a gatekeeper to shift from generic to client-specific assessment and treatment. The two orientations—medical necessity and clinical appropriateness—need to be reconciled and the conflicts resolved in order for a responsive, well-functioning managed care system to be designed, developed, and implemented.

Accountability

The fifth select issue is accountability. It focuses on identifying the best practice of patient care while also assessing the performance of treatment systems (Sederer & St. Clair, 1990; Zusman, 1988). There has been progress in measuring two initial indicators of quality—access and availability, and most managed care systems emphasize these two process or client satisfaction measures as their accountability measures. However, these have very little to do with true quality.

In fact, managed care gives little incentive to look at true quality. Through the incentive structure, practitioners are encouraged to attend to client satisfaction rather than the more difficult indicators of service quality—accurate diagnosis, proper intervention, and treatment impact. It is the last indicator, treatment impact, that is the most challenging for human service providers.

In larger part, attitudes toward accountability reflect a philosophical struggle about measuring an imprecise science and about the goals of intervention with people. If one takes a human potential perspective, then measurement is impossible. If one takes a goal-oriented perspective, then measurement is a professional responsibility. If one accepts the latter perspective, then there are some measures that the practice community can use to begin to address accountability. These measures include the quality of the patient's life, the patient's level of functioning, and the patient's symptom severity and medical cost offsets as they relate to employment, medical health, and psychological health. (For example: Is the patient going to work? Is the patient missing fewer days? Is treatment reducing other medical care costs?) Ultimately, we need to tie measures of quality to measures of both costs and savings. With these types of quality measurement, we should begin to see the best practices tied to cost. Chapter 9 describes one organization's effort to implement a system that can be held accountable for its services to the severely and profoundly mentally ill.

THE REST OF THE BOOK

The remainder of the book examines—through case examples and theoretical analyses—the implementation and impact of managed care in the human service context. The chapters discuss the implications of the designed managed care system at two of the three levels. Part 1 addresses system design and implementation. The four chapters illuminate, from different perspectives, managed care issues in the reconciliation of policy-level mandates and provider-level realities. Part 2 addresses the service provider network. The four case studies examine the service delivery experience under managed care—illustrating organizational planning, staff and customer expectations, financial and business arrangements, and collaboration, among other issues. Part 3 contains a conceptual analysis of the effect of managed care on the therapeutic relationship. The analyses and examples in this book come from the traditional social work fields of practice: child welfare, family services, and mental health. They describe how decisions at the (often state or national) policy level affect the system's design and ultimately the network of local service providers. They also show how the complex relationships and interinstitutional connections that exist in our system of human service provision will shape the design and implementation of managed care, and how managed care principles, in turn, will guide changes in our decentralized, and at times fragmented, approach to provision of human services.

Together the chapters of this book demonstrate how managed care is changing the field of social work and human services. The chapters sketch a picture of the new environment in which human service organizations operate and to which they must adapt in order to survive. The perspectives and conclusions of the contributors are mixed. Although there are many problems and challenges, the impact of managed care on the field of social work and human services is not all bad. As one CEO of a human service organization reflected, "Change was inevitable. Its name happened to be managed care."

REFERENCES

Abbott, B., Jordan, P., & Murtaza, N. (1995). Interagency collaboration for children's mental health services: The San Mateo County model for managed care. *Administration and Policy in Mental Health, 22*(3), 301–313.

Allen, D. W. (1993). Planning for the future of behavioral health services. *Health Care Strategic Management, 11*(10), 16–19.

Applebaum, R. A., & McGinnis, R. (1992). What price quality? Assuring the quality of case-managed in-home care. *Journal of Case Management, 1*(1), 9–13.

Behar, L. (1985). Changing patterns of state responsibility: A case study of North Carolina. *Journal of Clinical Child Psychology, 14*(3), 188–195.

Behar, L. (1990). Financing mental health services for children and adolescents. *Bulletin of the Menninger Clinic, 54*(1), 127–139

Belkin, L. (1996, December 8). But what about quality? *The New York Times Magazine,* pp. 68–71+.

Bickman, L. (1996). A continuum of care: More is not always better. *American Psychologist, 51*(7), 689–701.

Broskowski, A. (1991). Current mental health care environments: Why managed care is necessary. *Professional Psychology: Research and Practice, 22*(1), 6–14.

Christianson, J., & Gray, D. Z. (1994). What CMHC's can learn from two state's efforts to capitate Medicaid benefits. *Hospital and Community Psychiatry, 45*(8), 777–781.

Christianson, J. B., Manning, W., Lurie, N., Stoner, T. J., Gray, D. Z., Popkin, M., & Marriott, S. (1995). Utah's prepaid mental health plan: The first year *Health Affairs, 14*(3), 160–172.

Cole, R. E., Reed, S. K., Babigian, H. M., Brown, S. W., & Fray, J. (1994). A mental health capitation program: I. Patient outcomes. *Hospital and Community Psychiatry, 45*(11), 1090–1096.

Corcoran, K., & Vandiver, V. (1996). *Maneuvering the maze of managed care.* New York: Free Press.

DeLeon, P. H., VandenBos, G. R., & Bulatao, E. Q. (1991). Managed mental health care: A history of the federal policy initiative. *Professional Psychology: Research and Practice, 22*(1), 15–25.

Dorwart, R. A., & Schlesinger, M. (1988). Privatization of psychiatric services. *American Journal of Psychiatry, 145*(5), 543–553.

Feild, T. (1996, Summer). Managed care and child welfare. *Public Welfare*, pp. 4–10.

Fennell, M. L., & Alexander, J. A. (1993). Perspectives on organizational change in the U.S. medical care sector. *Annual Review of Sociology, 19*, 89–112.

Finkelstein, D. A., & Frissel, S. (1990). The systems/integrated approach to quality and cost-effective care. *Employee Assistance Quarterly, 61*(1), 25–43.

Frank, R. G., McGuire, T. G., & Newhouse, J. P. (1995). Risk contracts in managed mental health care. *Health Affairs, 14*(3), 50–64.

Freeborn, D. K., & Pope, C. R. (1994). *Promise and performance in managed care: The prepaid group practice model.* Baltimore: Johns Hopkins University Press.

Freund, D. A., & Hurley, R. E. (1995). Medicaid managed care: Contribution to issues of health reform. *Annual Review of Public Health, 16*, 473–495.

Golant, S. M., & McCasling, R. (1979). A functional classification of services for older people. *Journal of Gerontological Social Work, 1*(3), 187–209.

Goldstein, J. M. Bassuk, E. L., Holland, S. K., & Zimmer, D. (1988). Identifying catastrophic psychiatric cases: Targeting managed-care strategies. *Medical Care, 26*(8), 790–799.

Hicks, L. I., & Bopp, K. D. (1966). Integrated pathways for managing rural health services. *Health Care Management Review, 21*(1), 65–72.

Hoge, M. A., Davidson, L., Griffith, E. E. H., Sledge, W. H., & Howenstine, R. A. (1994). Defining managed care in public-sector psychiatry. *Hospital and Community Psychiatry, 45*(11), 1085–1089.

Hunter, A., Riger, S. (1986). The meaning of community in community mental health. *Journal of Community Psychology, 14,* 55–71.

Keigher, S. (1995). Managed care's silent seduction of America and the new politics of choice. *Health and Social Work, 20*(2), 146–151.

Levendusky, P. G., Willis, B. S., & Ghinassi, F. A. (1994). The therapeutic contracting program: A comprehensive continuum of care model. *Psychiatric Quarterly, 65*(3), 189–208.

Levin, B. L., Glasser, J. H., & Jaffee, C. L. (1986). National trends in coverage and utilization of mental health, alcohol, and substance abuse services within managed health care systems. *American Journal of Public Health, 78*(9), 1222–1223.

Martin, L., & Kettner, P. (1996). *Measuring the performance of human service programs.* Thousand Oaks, CA: Sage.

McGuire, T. G. (1994). Predicting the cost of mental health benefits. *Milbank Quarterly, 72*(1), 3–23.

Mechanic, D., Schlesinger, M., & McAlpine D. D. (1995). Management of mental health and substance abuse services: State of the art and early results. *Milbank Quarterly, 73*(1), 19–55.

Mordock, J. B. (1996). The road to survival revisited: Organizational adaptation to the managed care environment. *Child Welfare, 75*(3), 195–218.

Morrison Dore, M., Wilkerson, A. N., & Sonia, W. A. (1992). Exploring the relationship between a continuum of care and intrusiveness of children's mental health services. *Hospital and Community Psychiatry, 43*(1), 44–48.

Morrissey, J. P., & Goldman, H. H. (1986). Care and treatment of the mentally ill in the United States: Historical developments and reforms. *Annals of the American Political Science Society, 484,* 12–27.

Mullady, S. F. (1991). The Champion Paper Company EAP and major issues for employee assistance programs in the 1990s: Managed care and aging. *Employee Assistance Quarterly, 6*(3), 37–50.

Newman, L. (1995). Scrutinizing mental health outcomes: Behavioral outcomes systems redefine services and populations. *Managed Healthcare, 5*(9), 46.

Nyberg, D., & Marschke, P. (1993, Spring). Critical pathways: Tools for continuous quality improvement. *Nursing Administration Quarterly*, pp. 62–69.

Reed, S. K., Hennessy, K. D., Mitchell, O. S., & Babigian, H. M. (1994). A mental health capitation program: II Cost-benefit analysis. *Hospital and Community Psychiatry, 45*(11), 1097–1103.

Root, L. S. (1991). Cost controls on mental health services: Context and the role of the professional. *Employee Assistance Quarterly, 7*(2), 1–14.

Rothman, J. (1996). The interweaving of community intervention approaches. *Journal of Community Practice, 3*(3/4), 69–99.

Salamon, L. (1993). The marketization of welfare: Changing nonprofit and for-profit roles in the American welfare state. *Social Service Review, 67*(1), 16–39.

Schinnar, A. P., Rothbard, A. B., & Hadley, T. R. (1989). Opportunities and risks in Philadelphia's capitation financing of public psychiatric services. *Community Mental Health Journal, 25*(4), 255–266.

Schinnar, A. P., Rothbard, A. B., & Hadley, T. R. (1992). A prospective management approach to the delivery of public mental health services. *Administration and Policy in Mental Health, 19*(4), 291–308.

Sederer, L. I., & Bennett, M. J. (1996). Managed mental health care in the United States: A status report. *Administration and Policy in Mental Health, 23*(4), 289–306.

Sederer, L. I., & St. Clair, R. L. (1990). Quality assurance and managed mental health care. *Psychiatric Clinics of North America, 13*(1), 89–97.

Shortell, S., et al. (1996). *Remaking health care in America: Building organized delivery systems.* San Francisco: Jossey-Bass.

Spath, P. L. (1993). Critical paths: A tool for clinical process management. *Journal of American Health Information Management Association, 64*(3), 48–58.

Tuma, J. (1989). Mental health services for children: The state of the art. *American Psychologist, 44*(2), 188–199.

Watkins, J. M., Watkins, D. A. (1984). Continuum of care as a policy framework for the social/health care needs of the elderly: A state of the art review. *Journal of Gerontological Social Work, 6*(4), 49–64.

Webb, W. (19887). Ethical aspects of the continuum of care concept. *Psychiatric Hospital, 18*(4), 147–151.

Webber, H. S. (1995). The failure of health-care reform: An essay review. *Social Service Review, 69*(2), 309–322.

Winegar, N. (1993). Managed mental health care: Implications for administrators and managers of community-based agencies. *Families in Society: The Journal of Contemporary Human Services, 74*(3), 171–177.

Zusman, J. (1988). Quality assurance in mental health care. *Hospital and Community Psychiatry, 39*(12), 1286–1290.

PART ONE

Service System Design

The four chapters that follow discuss the structure of a managed care system. These chapters focus on the policy-making and the system design and implementation levels. In varying degrees, each chapter describes the elements of a managed care system within the classic social work practice arenas of child welfare or mental health.

Four themes emerge from these chapters. First, the demand for managed care in human services has evolved from the systems' failure to meet their legal mandates. Over the past thirty years human services systems have been charged with deinstitutionalizing their populations and implementing community-based services systems. Although the legal requirements have been met, achieving the spirit of the reforms has fallen far short. This failure is partly evidenced by jails and homeless shelters largely populated by the severely and profoundly mentally ill and turnstile placements of abused children. The current service system is fragmented, suffers from serious gaps, and provides few incentives to sustain service recipients in the community. As a result, the efficacy of the traditional human service systems that were established to serve and protect those citizens in greatest need is being called into question.

Second, multiple competing values and mandates will complicate, and perhaps prevent, implementation of managed care in public human services. For example, the debate between public goods and private responsibility is perennial and politicized, albeit clothed in cost-benefit and econometric vocabulary. Another conflict centers on the defined client. Is the client the individual (for example, a child who may be abused in which case the goal is to protect the child), or is it the family (in which case another goal is to protect the privacy of the family and minimize intrusion from the state)? Another conflict focuses on the treatment philosophy that undergirds the system. Is the focus on long-term service to chronic clients with multiple problems requiring continuous care, or is the focus on short-term service to clients with acute need? Yet another conflict pits privatization against public responsibility. Is a fully privatized system the best means of helping citizens in need? What roles does the public sector have in addressing the needs of its vulnerable citizens? Ultimately, only discourse and debate will resolve these issues.

Third, measurement is a glaring problem. Measurement takes numerous forms: outcomes, impact assessment, quality assurance, utilization review, and best practice. Our level of knowledge about service constellations is woefully inadequate. Little is known about which service mix works best with which constellation of client needs and problems. It is exceedingly difficult to assess quality and utilization when best practices are inadequately identified. Resources must be invested into measurement if outcome-oriented managed care is to be implemented successfully.

Fourth, cost savings are not guaranteed in a public human service system under managed care. As with "welfare reform," short-term savings may be procured in a redesigned system. However, like the newly designed "family assistance system" and physical health care systems, managed care in human service systems requires infusions of new resources from a variety of sources to ensure that an adequate and responsive system is being created.

Rycraft and Mordock discuss managed care in public child welfare. In chapter 2 Rycraft presents a historical and contextual analysis of managed care's relationship to child welfare. She discusses the inherent conflict between the mission of child welfare and the goals of managed care. She assesses the influence of the gatekeeping role and complex institutional relationship on system redesign. In particular, Rycraft highlights the role of the judiciary, a key actor often forgotten or neglected in these discussions and analyses.

Mordock, in chapter 3, discusses the early implementation of managed care in child welfare in the State of New York. He examines the impact of a multiple-provider policy on the system's design and implementation. He also addresses the historical experience of child welfare in a managed context. Mordock emphasizes the importance of information management, its role in system design and management, and the complex institutional relationships that constitute the child welfare system.

The impact of managed care on mental health systems has been explored in other publications. In chapter 4 Hudson explores the policy-making processes at the state level. His analysis focuses on the context of the first and second generations of mental health managed care in the Commonwealth of Massachusetts. The use and impact of a single-provider system achieved dollar savings but at considerable cost to the provider network. Further, the system did little to reduce service fragmentation. According to Hudson, the Massachusetts experiment did not pass the ultimate test for managed care in public human services—better services for those in greatest need.

Thomlison, Meade, and Prichard take up the focus on child welfare again in chapter 5. However, they present managed care from a Canadian perspective. This chapter depicts the inclusion of the community in the design of a comprehensive child and family service system (an approach to redesign and reinvention that is being adopted and introduced in the United States). The authors describe the difficulties in designing a community-based service delivery system. Their experience illustrates the need for a long-term perspective in both building and assessing the community-based continuum of care. This chapter also demonstrates the importance of a broad definition of quality as both system processes for citizen payers and system outcomes for clients.

Taken together, these chapters find mixed results for system redesign under managed care. There are some successes, some failures, and enormous challenges yet to be met. Bridging fragmented services as well as satisfying the complete interests of key participants will be great tasks in redesigning the public human service system. Public child welfare in particular will require inordinate investment of resources. Moreover, development of best practices and incorporation of all actors, especially the judiciary, may yet be the major hurdles to overcome.

CHAPTER 2

Challenges and Opportunities for Public Child Welfare

Joan R. Rycraft
AAF Assistant Professor, School of Social Work,
University of Texas at Arlington

Across the nation, media portrayals of the abandonment, deprivation, battering, molestation, and death of young children at the hands of their parents excite public outrage. Blame is placed not only on parents, but also on the public child welfare system, whose primary mandate is to protect children and preserve families. It is a system overwhelmed with increasing reports of child maltreatment, undermined by longstanding funding inadequacies, struggling with insufficient program resources, and in many areas lacking adequate professional staff. Moreover, it is under siege from the outside, facing massive litigation and ongoing media attacks, both signaling the need for substantive change. Today's child welfare service delivery system, called a "morass" by Courtney (1995), appears to have lost its direction, and few child welfare scholars or practitioners would disagree with Courtney's description. Highlighting major child welfare reform initiatives throughout history, this chapter will chronicle the evolution of the child welfare system up to the current movement to institute managed care principles and practices in the overall delivery of services. The crucial challenge to the successful implementation of managed care principles in child welfare services is the recognition that the philosophy, structure, goals, legal mandates, and span of autonomy in child welfare differ significantly from other social service systems that have developed a managed care model of service delivery. These unique aspects must be addressed when crafting a model of managed care for child welfare.

Child welfare programs are authorized through federal and state statutes. The statutes delineate eligibility for service benefits, determine fund-

The author expresses appreciation to Patricia Newlin, MSW, LMSW-ACP, University of Texas at Arlington, for her assistance in reviewing the managed care literature for this chapter.

ing mechanisms, and identify program administration responsibility. Each state must identify a single agency to operate its child welfare programs. Although an array of child welfare services are provided by not-for-profit, proprietary, and public sector institutions, the primary responsibility for programs and funding lies with a single state agency or local government agency under the supervision of the State (Stein, 1991).

Child welfare is a vast nationwide system made up of a continuum of services that encompasses investigation of child abuse and neglect reports, intensive services to prevent placement and preserve families, placement and maintenance of children in various levels of substitute care, preparation of adolescents for adult living, family reunification services, and adoption. It has developed into one of the largest, most complex social service systems in the nation.

Seemingly intractable social problems such as poverty, abuse and neglect, teen pregnancy, homelessness, substance abuse, and AIDS have become the domain of child welfare (Allen, 1991). Since the passage of the Child Abuse Prevention and Treatment Act in 1974, which mandated the reporting of suspected child maltreatment, reports of child abuse and neglect have nearly tripled. In 1994, the number of children reported as alleged victims of child abuse and neglect soared to almost 3 million (U.S. Department of Health and Human Services, National Center on Child Abuse and Neglect, 1996). On any given day, there are 85,000 children in need of adoption and 450,000 children living in foster care homes, group home care, and institutions (U.S. General Accounting Office, 1995). In the past decade, the monthly average number of children in substitute care increased 135.78%. Not surprisingly, the most significant increase occurred in states with large child populations—California, 145%; Florida, 302%; Illinois, 375%; New York, 181%; Pennsylvania, 130%; and Texas, 103%; (U.S. Department of Health and Human Services, Administration for Children and Family, 1996). Unquestionably, the current child welfare system is in crisis, unable to fully meet service demands, societal expectations, and its mandates of child protection and family preservation.

EVOLUTION OF THE CHILD WELFARE SYSTEM

Children were long viewed as the property of their parents with the father having absolute rights to their custody and control. However, as the specific needs of children became more apparent, as child populations decreased, and as enlightenment regarding the rights of all persons emerged, child rights also became an issue of concern. The history of child welfare, in its quest for child protection, is rich with notable movements toward providing the best casework practices of the time. Through the child-saving era of the seventeenth century, the child-rescue era of the early nineteenth century, and the historic first White House Conference on Children in 1909, significant changes have occurred in the services provided to children and their families. From a local system of caring for dependent children through indenture and institutional housing, to rescuing children from the pitfalls of urban strife and transplanting them to rural midwestern foster homes, the plight of dependent children was eventually brought to the attention of the nation. During the latter part of the nineteenth century, childhood came to be viewed as a special time of life and children were recognized as having rights that included access to education, provision of basic needs such as food, shelter, and clothing, and protection from too early labor, immoral influences, and physical abuse. Basic societal norms regarding childhood and child rearing slowly developed, and legal measures were eventually taken to ensure that children's rights would be protected. This emerging relationship between the state and families and children was formalized with the creation of the juvenile court at the end of the nineteenth century (Cohen, 1992; Stein, 1991).

Juvenile court is a state institution charged with the responsibility of balancing families' rights to privacy and the state's mandate to protect children and their rights. The purview of state intervention into family life has long been and continues to be debated by legal scholars. Individual state statutes specify the authority of the court, with jurisdiction in most states extending to minors charged with legal violations and dependent children who have been abused, neglected, or abandoned. Juvenile court should be viewed as a gatekeeper within the continuum of child welfare services. The ultimate decisions regarding child protection, out-of-home placement, and family preservation and reunification are the domain of the juvenile court and its presiding judge.

The 1909 White House Conference on Children issued the resolution that children should remain in their homes if there are no "urgent or compelling" reasons for their removal and recommended the establishment of a Children's Bureau. With the creation of the Children's Bureau in 1912, the federal government formally entered the field of child welfare services. The passage of the Social Security Act of 1935 established the foundation of our current social service system. Title V of the Social Security Act addressed social service needs of abandoned, abused, and neglected children. Additionally, grants were made available to all states and territories through the Children's Bureau to develop child welfare services (Cohen, 1992; Morton, 1993).

During the next twenty-five years, child welfare services expanded through provision of concrete services to maintain children in their homes and a growing use of foster care homes for those children who could not remain in the parental home. Anecdotal, historical reports draw a vivid picture of increasing numbers of children living in parental homes described as dysfunctional and disorganized and being placed in foster care for their safety and protection. These children were reported as having serious problems resulting in long stays in foster care, with many never returning to the parental home. It appeared that more and more children were entering and growing to adulthood in foster care. A 1959 landmark study conducted by the Child Welfare League of America (CWLA) found a dismal disarray of services provided to children placed in foster care and their families. Children were being removed simply because their families were poor and for other questionable reasons; minority and poor children were overrepresented in the foster care population; and little, if any, emphasis was placed on returning children to the parental home. Once removed, children were provided few services, and their families almost none (Maas & Engler, 1959). Based on these findings, CWLA put forth an urgent call to curtail the unnecessary placement of children in substitute care. Standards were developed that identified home-based services as preferred services provided to children and families. The call went unheeded, and subsequent research supported Maas and Engler's earlier findings. Children were being placed in substitute care at increasing rates. Once placed, children drifted from home to home until they reached the age of majority and then were dismissed from the system.

Kempe's coining of the term "battered child syndrome" in the early 1960s is viewed as society's "rediscovery" of child abuse (1962). This medical diagnosis based on forensic review of children's bone fracture x-rays brought the problem of child abuse to the attention of the general public. The medical community began to recognize the pervasiveness of nonaccidental injuries to children at the hands of their caretakers. As reports of child abuse increased and became publicized through the media, the issue of child maltreatment became a target for politicians seeking an innovative agenda. Senator Walter Mondale (D-MN) and Representative Patricia Schroeder (D-CO) were key players in the passage of the Child Abuse Prevention and Treatment Act of 1974 (CAPTA, PL 93–247). The focus of this legislation was funding for demonstration projects to prevent, identify, and treat child abuse and neglect. It also created the National Center on Child Abuse and Neglect, a clearinghouse for information on child maltreatment. Eligibility for CAPTA funding required states to establish procedures for the reporting of suspected child maltreatment. The nationwide response to this legislation was the passing of state laws that include mandatory reporting procedures and definitions of child maltreatment. Although well intentioned, this legislation has been harshly criticized as exacerbating the problems of a system already in failure:

> The law fails to specify the conditions that should be defined as child abuse or neglect or the evidential standards for reporting. Moreover, although the intent of the legislation is conveyed clearly in its title, the implementing regulations focused attention on mandatory reporting and investigation, not prevention and treatment. Consequently, this law has had the effect of greatly enlarging the pool of children coming to the attention of public authorities as potentially in need of care and protection, without providing the resources or guidelines necessary to enable states to deal more effectively with this population. (McGowan, 1990, p. 72)

Following enactment of the legislation, reports of suspected child maltreatment quickly overran the capabilities of the child welfare system. The system was already the target of criticism due to its lack of effective service delivery and large numbers of children were experiencing foster care drift.

In response to the explosion in the numbers of children coming into the system and criticisms of foster care programs, major reforms were passed at the federal level. These reform efforts were crafted on the principle of providing permanency for all children entering the child welfare system. The Adoption Assistance and Child Welfare Act of 1980 (PL 96–272) mandated specific programs and practices to ensure "reasonable efforts" to prevent placement and detailed plans to provide permanent living situations for children placed in substitute care. With a goal of permanency for every child, casework practices were to be individualized and targeted toward returning children to their parents or, if reunification was not feasible, freeing them for adoption or maintaining them in long-term placements.

There have, however, been myriad difficulties in implementing the reforms, causing some critics to denounce the permanency planning movement. As has become customary with social service programs, many of the mandates were underfunded, leaving states scrambling to meet the costs of the new requirements. In addition to a substantial lack of financial support, another explosion of reports of child abuse and neglect occurred due partly to a national epidemic of crack and cocaine use. Presently, children coming into the system are much younger (George, Wulczyn, & Harden, 1995), staying in placement longer (Barth, Courtney, Duerr Berrick, & Albert, 1994), and showing severe problems (English, Allen, & DeWoody, 1994).

Additionally, the emphasis on placement prevention has actually thwarted efforts to move children out of care and reunify them with their families. Throughout the nation, child welfare agencies target more resources for family preservation services and foster care than for family reunification efforts. Family reunification programs are viewed as costly with low rates of success. An ongoing decline in the rate of children leaving substitute care has influenced the growth of substitute care nationwide and brings the efficacy of permanency planning into question (Tatara, 1994).

These two major legislative directives—PL 96–272, with its principle of permanency planning and CAPTA, with its mandate of child abuse and neglect reporting—appear to create a paradox in child welfare policy and practice (Jimenez, 1990). Compliance with CAPTA mandates brings larger numbers of children into the system, while PL 96–272 was enacted to provide permanency to children, preferably within their parental homes. Added to this confusion is the Family Preservation and Support Act of 1993. Advocates of family preservation fought a long, hard battle to ensure financial support of programs that emphasize preventing placements and preserving families. A plethora of studies evaluating family preservation programs have provided substantial data for both sides of the debate regarding the efficacy of family preservation. For every study that reports high success rates of preventing placement is another study that indicates otherwise.

In reviewing the historical evolution of the current child welfare system, an argument can be made that children and their families are somewhat better served today. Although the preservation of children and families and permanency planning are the current guiding principles of child welfare services, warranted criticisms continue as successful outcomes for families are scarce and incidents of child abuse and neglect escalate.

SEARCH FOR SUCCESSFUL INTERVENTIONS AND PREVENTION

To date, there are no definitive validated "best practices" for the prevention and treatment of child maltreatment, nor is there agreement on desired outcomes for children and families. A major challenge to defining measurable outcomes in child welfare is the unrealistic expectations held by the general public. By design, default, devilish dream, or divine intervention, the public expects the child welfare system to prevent child abuse and neglect, eradicate poverty, transform parents, and, if unable to do so, make necessary arrangements to ensure that all children are raised in happy, healthy families. No matter that these expectations are totally unrealistic, it is the reality of child welfare today. Underlying these expectations is the prevailing belief that the primary cause of child maltreatment is parents' behavior. This view ignores any socioenvironmental factors. Commonly known as the "medical model," this approach to child maltreatment "fits the quintessential American view of all social problems, they are individually rooted, described as an illness, and solvable by occasional doses of therapeutic conversation" (Nelson as cited in Wexler, 1995, p. 56).

The present child welfare service delivery system is built on the medical model despite overwhelming evidence of a link between poverty and child maltreatment (Wexler, 1995). Child welfare scholars posit that if poverty were eradicated, reports of child maltreatment could decline by 50% (Pecora, Whittaker, & Maluccio, 1992), and if social workers concentrated on providing preventive and income support services to families, the numbers of children placed in substitute care would be reduced (Lindsey, 1994). Although these statements have not been empirically validated, there is evidence that poverty is a major contributing factor in child abuse and neglect. However, poverty also is viewed as a result of individual apathy, laziness, and dependence, thus again placing responsibility and blame on the individual parent. In essence, society refuses to take any responsibility for many of its most serious problems. Thus, "whenever problems which are actually rooted in societal dynamics are defined as individual pathology or shortcomings, their real sources are disguised, interventions are focused on individuals . . . and the social order is absolved by implication from guilt and responsibility and may continue to function unchallenged in accordance with established patterns" (Gil, 1981, p. 312).

Upon this foundation, children and families brought to the attention of the child welfare system for incidents of child maltreatment are separated under the auspices of child protection. The children are placed into substitute care and the parents, more often than not, are subjected to therapy and parent training programs. Services address the individual behavior identified as the "cause" of the maltreatment. Blaming individuals or society does not resolve the problems of families coming into the child welfare system.

Repeated efforts to reform the child welfare system over the past quarter of a century have for the most part produced only unrealized expectations and "broken promises" (Grubb & Lazarson, 1982). The failure of reforms has been attributed to the continuing tension between child and parental rights, society's inclination to provide only basic support for families, emphases on procedure, rules, and regulations rather than service provision, unrealistic public expectations of the system, the severity of the problems of the children and families in the system, and pervasive poverty (McGowan, 1991). We continue with a system that is residual, fragmented, and constrained in its archaic approach (Sarri & Finn, 1992).

Central to any substantive reform effort in child welfare practice is some resolution of the continuing debate between children's rights and rights of families to their privacy and child-rearing practices. Although the general public professes to strongly support the protection of children from abuse and neglect, there is little agreement about what actually constitutes abuse and neglect or when it is appropriate or acceptable for the state to intervene in family life. Societal norms vary among communities in regard to child-rearing practices. What may be seen as acceptable in one community may be viewed as abusive or neglectful in another. Our society's strong belief in individualism and privacy is in direct opposition to state intervention in personal activities such as child rearing. Although agreement that intervention is warranted is easily found in such egregious situations as child torture, rape, and murder, the vast majority of incidents reported to child welfare fall into a shady area requiring the application of laws that are fraught with ambiguity. For every person who believes the state should intervene in a particular situation is another who disagrees. Until the rights and protection of children are balanced with or possibly supersede the rights of family privacy, the child welfare system must continue to deal with ambiguities and constant questioning of its mandate and authority.

Despite earnest reform efforts, the child welfare system is viewed as an exorbitantly costly failure. Reports of child abuse and neglect continue to rise; despite casework efforts in family preservation the number of children in out-of-home care is escalating; children are coming into the system at young ages and staying longer periods of time; and thousands of children await adoptive homes. The fiscal costs of this failure are increasing at an alarming rate. The societal costs are incalculable.

FINANCING OF CHILD WELFARE

The funding mechanisms for child welfare services are as complex and varied as the program and services provided. States cover the major costs for foster care services and other child welfare services. The federal government, however, shares a substantial portion of the burden, approximately $4.1 billion in 1995 (U.S. General Accounting Office, 1995). The major source of funding for the child welfare system comes from Titles IV-E and IV-B of the Social Security Act, with smaller amounts from Titles XX and IV-A. Title IV-E, an open-ended entitlement of funds, covers the costs of foster care maintenance (supervision, shelter, food, clothing, etc.) of children from AFCE-eligible families and adoption assistance to families adopting "special needs" children. It also covers specific "administrative costs" incurred by the states to implement foster care services and provides training funds for child welfare staff. A growing number of states have developed collaborative partnerships with schools of social work for the enhancement of child welfare workers' knowledge and skills through social work degree programs and continuing education training. Title IV-B is a capped appropriation to cover child welfare services, which include foster care services and family preservation and support services to children remaining in their homes. Title XX funds are received through a social service block grant with disbursement determined by states and local entities. The actual amount of Title XX funds allocated to child welfare services is unknown. However, the recent 15% reduction in Title XX appropriations all but guarantees a comparable, if not greater, reduction of those funds allocated to child welfare services. Title IV-A emergency assistance funds are claimed to cover preventive services, family preservation, and counseling of at-risk families.

In addition, several states claim Title XIX Medicaid funds for provision of "medical services" provided by substitute care providers (U.S. General Accounting Office, 1995; Woodard, 1996). Most medical services and behavioral health services provided to children and families in the child welfare system are funded through Medicaid. Every child entering out-of-home care must have a medical and dental screening. Many of the children and their parents are referred for psychological testing and ongoing mental health services. All of these services are funded through Medicaid for every eligible person. To meet this increase in service need, throughout the country managed care companies have entered the behavioral health field. Doty (1996) reports that "in the last few years over 40 states have applied for and/or begun to implement either statewide or local 'Medicaid Managed Care' waiver programs" (p. 4).

Public assistance programs are also connected to the child welfare system. Most children and families reported to child welfare are receiving or have received some type of public assistance. Child care funding is a necessity for most parents to escape the public assistance cycle. It is not yet known what impact the 1996 welfare reform initiatives will have on the child welfare system but every implemented waiver contains funding for child care and medical services. In addition to children reported as abused or neglected, child welfare funding also covers children who are developmentally disabled or diagnosed as mentally ill, runaway youth, and juveniles placed in correctional facilities. Federal and state funding for this vast array of children and family programs and services continues to increase, yet the problems remain unresolved.

The largest share of funding supports substitute care maintenance costs primarily through purchase-of-service contracts with placement agencies and administrative costs of the placing agency (a state or local government child welfare agency). The current system has fiscal incentives that can entice substitute care providers to behave counter to the system's goals. In most states there is a hierarchal system of substitute care with commensurate rates of compensation. Placement agencies receive higher rates of compensation for children requiring intensive supervision and specialized treatment services. When program services are successful, the children eventually require less supervision and a lower level of service, at which time payment rates are lowered. However, the costs of running these programs do not decrease proportionately with each individual child who requires a lower level of service. For example, a child requiring intensive supervision and treatment may be placed in a program for a cost of $3,000 per month. During the next six months of care, the child's behavior improves to the point that the level of service can be reduced to care that is compensated at the lower rate of $2,000. Thus the placement agency continues to care for the child at a reduced rate even though the overall actual costs of the placement borne by the agency have not diminished by the same amount. In some instances, "success" can result in a loss of total funding for the child through reunification with his or her family, or removal from the agency to one that offers the appropriate level of care at a lower cost. As with medical facilities, the fiscal health of placement agencies is directly linked to the number of occupied beds. With multiple "successes" the agency may lose substantial funding. For financial survival, agencies are placed in the position of maintaining children at the highest level of supervision and treatment rather than encouraging a lower level of care or a return to home.

Despite reform efforts to prevent placements, substitute care costs have increased at an alarming rate over the past ten years. Nationally, federal foster care expenditures increased 242% between 1984 and 1995. These expenditures cover maintenance, administration, training, and state informational system costs. Of particular note are the proportionate decrease in maintenance costs and increase in administrative costs. The share of maintenance costs have dropped from 61.5% in 1988 to 52.3% in 1995. Average administrative monthly costs per case are 39.78% of total expenditures nationwide and actually exceed maintenance costs in twenty states. This provides some support to the notion that it is the administration costs of public agencies that are driving the cost of child welfare services to unacceptable levels, in other words, that the government's running of the system is a major source of the problem of spiraling costs. In the past three years, there have also been significant increases in Title IV-A emergency assistance expenditures. Caseloads have increased from 54,979 in 1993 to 80,034 in 1995, with a per case expenditure increase from $2,112 to $3,386. Total Title IV-A costs increased in this three-year period from $788,668 to $3,251,687 (U.S. Department of Health and Human Services, Administration for Children and Families, 1996).

All projections indicate a continued increase in the number of children entering the child welfare system and escalating costs for their care. Child welfare has become big business and can no longer be administered as an informal local social service system. In this era of accountability and cost containment, critics are calling for drastic measures ranging from total dismantling and restructuring to complete privatization of the system.

PRIVATIZATION IN CHILD WELFARE

The issue of privatization is integral to the provision of child welfare services. Historically, child welfare was the domain of private volunteer agencies. The government sector did not enter the field and provide funding until the early 1900s. It was the private sector that established the Societies for the Protection of Children. The Child Welfare League of America was initiated to provide standards and supportive services to the growing number of private volunteer agencies serving children and families.

With the expansion of the child welfare service system, large numbers of voluntary, not-for-profit agencies have been granted purchase-of-service contracts by governmental agencies. These private agencies continue to be substantial providers of child welfare services. In some areas, private agencies provide the majority of services to children and families. A transition from a mixed delivery system to a completely privatized approach has recently occurred. Kansas has been "the first state to privatize the administration and delivery of child welfare services" (Strausbaugh & Drissel, 1997). Texas is currently engaging in a pilot project that will privatize out-of-home care services in one region of the state (J. Woodard, ACF Region VI, personal communication, August 8, 1997).

Brodkin and Young (1989) present a cogent discussion of the political economy of privatization. Musgrave states that the primary role of government is the 1) distribution of wealth, 2) allocation of resources, and 3) stabilization of the economy (as cited in Brodkin & Young, 1989). The distribution of wealth is particularly germane to the privatization debate. He posits that if the government reduces its services to the poor, financial inequalities between the wealthy and the poor will be exacerbated. The marketplace will be then called upon to accept the task of distributing wealth through charitable giving. Historically, charitable giving has not been able to meet escalating needs. The result has been increased government supports with requisite regulations.

Salamon views the current prevalence of purchase-of-service contracts employed in child welfare as a "partnership that overcomes the problems of direct government provision and elements of voluntary failure" (as cited in Brodkin & Young, 1989, p. 134). These contractual agreements, however, can pose problems. Williamson notes that the small numbers of potential service providers and the practice of contract renewal with established providers may limit access by other providers (as cited in Brodkin & Young, 1989). This situation exists in many communities where one or two established not-for-profit social service agencies have held the child welfare purchase-of-service contracts for several years. Even when the need for services increases, the established contracts are often enlarged, thus continuing to limit competition for the potentially lucrative contracts.

Every part of the service sector—government, voluntary or not-for-profit, and proprietary—has both strengths and weaknesses to bring to the provision of services. Based on economic theories "various arrangements and combinations of profit-making, nonprofit, and public organizations may be seen as niches into which different goods and services fit so as to provide those goods and services in the most efficient way" (Brodkin & Young, 1989, p. 139), and an economist would probably suggest privatization as a way to improve efficiency in the provision of services. Privatization of child welfare service delivery, however, is an issue not only of efficiency but of policy and politics. Politically, privatization is seen as a means to control the growth of governmental bureaucracies and increase the role of communities in service provision. With the recent passage of welfare reform, and other plans to cut costs of public services on the table, privatization will certainly continue and probably escalate.

Although privatization is not a major change in child welfare service delivery, there is a call for substantive change in funding methods. Seeking a more efficient and effective service delivery system, child welfare is entering another era of reform. The most widely used and increasingly lauded method of service provision is managed care. Managed care has been promoted as an administratively sound system of quality assessment and cost containment in the appropriate distribution of social services. Following in the footsteps of other social service delivery systems, child welfare is preparing for its entrance into the arena of managed care (Feild, 1996).

THE MANAGED CARE MOVEMENT IN CHILD WELFARE

Although managed care is not a new concept in service delivery, there is little empirical evidence to date that it delivers on its promise of cost containment and service efficiency and efficacy. Critics contend that managed care may actually prevent access to needed services while increasing profits for management systems. Advocates maintain that unnecessary services are eliminated and appropriate services are targeted to specific populations, thus reducing overall costs. While the debate continues, child welfare administrators across the nation are designing a variety of models with a primary focus on cost containment and measurable service outcomes. This newest reform effort has emerged slowly and considerable planning appears to be taking place to ensure its success.

A nationwide survey of child welfare agencies, conducted by CWLA, indicated that managed care was a topic of interest in almost every state. Eighty-two percent of the states have already adopted or are considering applying managed care principles to child welfare financing and service delivery. Although there is wide variation across the states, a restructuring of child welfare administration and practices is the major change being considered. Potential changes include total state responsibility for integrated services, state oversight with contracts for specific management functions, and contracts with both not-for-profit and for-profit organizations for carved-in and carved-out service delivery. For example:

> Illinois is developing regional service bureaus with comprehensive case-management for children in out-of-home placements, local area provider networks and multi provider networks between child mental health and child welfare provider organizations. The overall goal is for these networks to function as management service or managed care organizations. Massachusetts is issuing [requests for proposals] for services for adolescents in state custody with capitation rates on funding. The intention is to award contracts to several agencies for service provision and one agency for service management. Michigan has a pilot project which uses a combination of Title IV-A and Medicaid funds to purchase services. The contract is pre-paid with capitated rates. Ohio has initiated a collaboration between public and private agencies to form an administrative services organization to manage funds. The funds have been pooled or integrated from several service systems (mental health, child welfare etc.). The funds are earmarked for children and adolescents placed in out-of-home care and paid under a capitated rate. (Doty, 1996)

Most changes currently planned are to be introduced incrementally for targeted populations, limited geographic regions, and specific services. The deflection from substitute care such as family foster care, group care, and residential treatment is the specific goal targeted in most managed care plans. Stated overall goals for managed care include higher quality of services, cost efficiency, and increased client satisfaction (McCullough, 1996c). It is not surprising that out-of-home care services are the focus of most managed care initiatives. As noted before, the largest cost within the child welfare service delivery system is the administration and maintenance of out-of-home care. Successful interventions in this arena will give the greatest return. Fewer children in care and shorter lengths of stay in care will reduce costs significantly, freeing funds for more placement prevention and prevention of child abuse and neglect.

Inevitably, the effort to adopt managed care principles in the administration and delivery of services will face challenges and problems. A definitive model for managed care in child welfare has yet to emerge. As states move into more planning for the introduction of managed care principles into child welfare service delivery and administration, it is important that mechanisms for utilization review and quality assurance be integral elements of the reform.

Cost containment and potential savings, targeted service delivery of a contin-uum of care, and successful outcomes will need to be documented. Medical services have been under managed care for several years, albeit with mixed reviews, and child welfare will most likely have its share of failures and suc-cesses also as it moves to a full-scale managed care system. Success of a man-aged care system depends on sound planning, adequate funding, and consis-tent implementation. "No successful managed care conversion has ever occurred without sufficient start-up funding and a complete array of high-quality technical and human resource tools" (McCullough, 1996a, p. 1). In several states the planning has begun; the elements of funding and imple-mentation will need to be in place also if this reform is to benefit the children and families in the child welfare system.

MANAGED CARE ELEMENTS

The emphasis of managed care is on an integrated system that manages financial risk under capitation (Authier, 1996). In order to achieve this goal in a managed care welfare system, several elements are essential. These include system design, capitation and performance contracting, preauthorization and gatekeeping, and utilization review.

System Design

There are numerous potential configurations for a managed care system in child welfare. The overall design should be carefully crafted based on pro-jected service needs, service utilization, available resources, and program goals and desired outcomes.

In most states and many communities the service delivery system is made up of a number of small and large private not-for-profit social service agencies that provide an array of child welfare services. Under almost any managed care system there is a strong potential that there will eventually be fewer but larger service provider agencies. In managed behavioral care, for example, nine or ten large, nationally managed care organizations control over 90% of the market (Doty, 1996). To maintain viability many smaller agencies will need to arrange partnerships in which they can pool capital, share finan-cial risks, cover a broader geographical area, and provide a wider array of ser-vices. There is also concern that if corporate managed care organizations are allowed to enter the child welfare service delivery system, the community ser-vice network that has been built over several decades will disappear. Unable to compete, small agencies will be forced out of service delivery. In the event that the corporate entity withdraws, because fiscal incentives are lacking or for other reasons, communities will have lost a local service system that took many years to develop and will have nothing to take its place. Each state must decide what configuration will best serve its client population now and in the future. Care must be taken not to dismantle or endanger the positive aspects of the existing delivery system in the quest to design a new potentially more cost-efficient and accountable system.

As previously noted, out-of-home care administrative costs are escalating. Emphasis is currently being placed on cost containment of substitute care services, which include family foster care, group home care, and residential treatment facilities. There are anecdotal reports of private not-for-profit agencies entering into agreements with state child welfare agencies to provide specific substitute care services with funding maintained at the current level of capitated rate. This activity reflects the belief that private agencies can provide high-quality services at lower cost than governmental agencies. Success in these efforts has yet to be determined and reported; however, historically there has been consistent evidence that private agencies are successful in high-quality, less costly service provision.

Although substitute care may be a good place to start designing a managed care system, control of the entry point to child welfare will eventually have to be addressed. Child protective services are the gatekeeper of the child welfare system. Children are not placed in substitute care without first going through a child protective services investigation. If attention is given only to substitute care services, a problematic imbalance may be created between contained last-end services and uncontained front-end services. Thus the state agency and the private agency provider must collaborate to balance between child protective services and all other service components within the child welfare system.

Equally important is the determination of current and projected utilization of services. How many children are currently in substitute care? How many children referred to child protective services are expected to be placed in substitute care, and at what level of care? How many families are receiving or projected to receive family preservation services? How many adoptions are completed annually, and how many children are still awaiting adoption? In designing a managed care system in child welfare, this information is necessary to guide decisions about service provision and adequate funding for contracted services.

Contrary to popular belief, the introduction of managed care does not necessarily result in a decrease in services. It should, however, result in a clear articulation of what services are to be provided, to whom, when, and at what cost. The delivery system must provide services to an identified population based on clear projections of service need and of costs of providing the services, including historical data and actuarial estimates on service use and cost. Such projection may be very difficult for child welfare. Child welfare does not control the factors that bring children and families to its door. For example, when public welfare reform goes into effect, a backlash on child welfare could be created. Forced from public assistance with no employment income, families will not be able to adequately care for their children thus creating massive demand for child welfare to place the children in substitute care. Added to this is the historically poor record keeping within child welfare, which will hinder attempts to determine service utilization and project service needs. Also, the open-ended allocation of Title IV-E substitute care funds has assured states that when projected costs are exceeded, additional funds will be available. Under managed care, this may not be the case. Agencies providing these services will need to develop mechanisms to track service need and utilization carefully or they will face fiscal disaster.

A final consideration in designing the system is identifying the agency that will manage the system, determine service providers, and address linkage between child welfare and other service systems such as the juvenile or family court, juvenile justice, and mental health. With its legal mandate of child protection, the state public child welfare agency is unlikely to completely relinquish its overall management of the system. Unless laws are rewritten, the public child welfare agency will continue to be the gatekeeper to child welfare services through child protective services investigations. It is conceivable, however, that more states will follow Kansas and have public child welfare provide only child protection investigation services and privatize all other services under a managed care service design.

Capitation and Performance Contracting

Child welfare agencies and their ancillary service providers have become dependent on the categorical funding mechanisms of federal programs. Under managed care, funding will change from purchase-of-service contracting to capitated rates.

Little attention has been paid to the true costs of child welfare services. If service costs are not calculated correctly, an agency runs the risk of substantial fiscal loss. Most voluntary social service agencies exist on shoestring budgets, and it is unlikely that they can absorb large financial losses. To set correct capitated rates, the type of service and its true cost, based on historical and projected service utilization, must be identified. For example, the true cost of substitute care includes more than simply foster care maintenance payments to foster parents or to a placement facility. The full cost of services include administrative overhead, salaries and benefits of staff implementing the program, management staff, and a determined allowance for unexpected or unusually high costs.

To control financial risk, a variety of payment options can be considered. These include contract incentives, under which agencies are given financial inducement to reduce the actual cost of services; no-risk outcome-driven contracts, which allow full funding even if an innovative intervention is unsuccessful and provide opportunities to refine interventions for positive outcomes; and carve-outs that exclude specific target populations, such as severely emotionally disturbed adolescents, from the service contract. Another option is performance contracting, which joins purchase-of-service contracting with capitation. Providers receive a block of start-up costs, partial payment for delivered services, and a balloon payment on successful outcome after the end of the contract. Whichever method is selected, all parties must understand clearly the inclusions and exclusions in payment for services.

Preauthorization and Gatekeeping

Although the financial aspect of risk management is important, vigilance for harm to a vulnerable population must be paramount. Under managed care, the type and amount of service to be provided are determined by a case manager who is not the actual service provider. The person making decisions about care provision will not have personal knowledge of clients and their individual needs and may not have the professional experience or education of the direct service provider. This creates tension between the managed care gatekeeper or case manager and the highly trained professionals who are requesting approval of service provision. For social workers this transition is often difficult as they no longer have full discretion regarding client case plans.

In the child welfare arena, the decisions made by the managed care gatekeeper can have disastrous effects on a child. If a child welfare caseworker is told that a child does not qualify for placement, or if a placement agency refuses to place a child as requested by the child welfare caseworker, the child will have to remain in a home that may have high potential for harm. Should that child be injured or harmed, who will be held accountable? Whether the managed care program will accept accountability is the subject of great debate. The child welfare agency will hesitate to assign decision-making activities to another system if that system will not be held responsible and liable for its decisions.

The child welfare agency can also be placed in an untenable position between the juvenile court and the managed care system. If a judge orders placement and the managed care case manager denies the request for services, the child welfare agency is placed in a position of noncompliance with a court order. Professionals who have worked with the juvenile court system will appreciate the difficulties of this situation for the caseworker and child welfare agency. In yet another scenario, the managed care system may determine that a child no longer needs to be in substitute care and can be returned home, yet to do so, the child welfare caseworker must obtain a court order. If the judge does not agree with the plan to return the child to the parental home, the child welfare agency will again be placed in an impossible position.

Clearly, there must be some method of redress built into the system design. Specific safeguards must be in place to prevent inappropriate denial of services or substandard service delivery that may place a child at risk. The State of Texas recently passed legislation allowing litigation against health maintenance organizations and other managed care operations for denial of services. Although this is certainly one avenue of redress, if a child is denied services and is subsequently harmed, the legal system will only be dealing with the situation after the fact.

Utilization Review

Several aspects of managed care are subsumed under utilization review. These include service array, provider network, job functions, information management, and outcomes.

Child welfare provides a standard and limited array of services that include parent training, day care, substitute care, monitoring, and counseling. Service provision must cover the child and the family, with each member often needing a different mix of services. A major concern in child welfare is that little evidence exists that substantiates significant, longitudinal impact of services. For the most part services are designed to change behavior and do not address the underlying causes for the behavior. The linkages between assessment, treatment, and outcomes are unclear or are not addressed in any systematic form. Moving into managed care without a clear definition of improved provision of services may initially lower costs, but it is doubtful that outcomes will be significantly better. Needed are accepted standards of practice delineating specific interventions and their utilization, decision-making protocols that provide guidelines and processes to be followed in determining who receives services and the type of services, and systematic case reviews to ensure consistent quality.

The capability and quality of the service providers is pivotal to the success of a managed care system. Current service providers must be evaluated to determine their qualifications, staffing competency, fiscal stability, and ability to perform under a managed care program. Criteria must be established, and procedures developed, to assess the strengths and limitations of potential service providers. To assure fairness, agreed upon grievance procedures and an appeals process will also need to be developed and implemented.

Utilization management will place the child welfare agency in the position of closely monitoring contracts and providing fewer casework services. This will require substantive changes in job functions with requisite training. The vast majority of staff in child welfare agencies are trained to be caseworkers not contract monitors. Child welfare administrators are trained in social work not in business activities. Another consideration is that since child welfare's inception, staff turnover has been a major administrative issue. An often cited reason for leaving child welfare is the lack of opportunity to use professional education and skills in the treatment of children and families. Under a managed care system that will emphasize contract monitoring, continuing turnover of experienced caseworkers should be expected.

Information management is a necessary element in developing and maintaining an efficient and effective managed care system. Decisions made regarding utilization, service provision, and profit and loss require accurate and current information. Management information systems in child welfare are archaic, impossible to refine, or fragmented beyond ability to interface. At best they provide questionable or unstable information; at worst they are nonexistent. Few agencies can provide accurate counts of children and families receiving services or the type and amount of services being provided. In response to continued and strong requests from the states and child welfare administrators, scholars, and advocates, Congress appropriated funds to design and maintain state automated child welfare information systems. These systems will together become a cornerstone of the effort to provide utilization data necessary to successfully manage child welfare programs. Until a workable information system is in place, implementation of managed care practices may be premature.

The greatest challenge facing child welfare practice is determining measurable outcomes for children and families in the areas of child safety, family connectedness, and child and family well-being. For the most part, child welfare agencies have yet to focus on service effectiveness or develop tools to evaluate the efficacy of services. Basic outcomes for any managed care system include 1) whether agreed upon services were rendered, 2) whether clients benefitted from the services as intended, and 3) whether the services provided were cost efficient. If designed and implemented appropriately, an outcome management system should identify the type of clients who were treated successfully and determine the most and least successful interventions. Case plans will have to be outcome oriented with measurable behavioral indicators, target dates, and systematic monitoring of client functioning. Additionally, levels of satisfaction of all players—for example, payers, providers, consumers, and the courts—must be assessed. A managed care system may show cost efficiency, but without consumer satisfaction there has been nothing but a fiscal gain. In the human service arena, the "bottom line" must be a combination of client satisfaction and fiscal integrity.

Managed care requires concurrent utilization review. All services and their associated costs must be monitored during the life of each case. Continuous monitoring is necessary to ensure efficiency, cost containment, and effectiveness. The tracking of cases and service delivery must address the services, the costs, and the delivery system's operation. Procedures will also need to be introduced that identify those situations outside the control of the service provider that may affect utilization, such as court decisions, policy changes, and legislative mandates.

CHALLENGES TO IMPLEMENTATION OF MANAGED CARE IN CHILD WELFARE

Child welfare nationwide is embarking on another reform effort in its search for an efficient and effective service delivery system. Following in the footsteps of physical and behavioral health care, various elements of the child welfare system are being redesigned under managed care principles and practices. Although the physical and behavioral health care system and the child welfare system have many similarities, unique aspects of child welfare should be considered in the process of implementing managed care.

Philosophy and Legal Mandate

Child welfare service delivery is based on the principles of protection and permanency, neither of which may be served by time-limited service provision. The range of responsibility placed on the child welfare system far outreaches those of the mental or physical health care system. Nor does child welfare have the right to refuse to provide services. In other words, child welfare is mandated to provide all necessary services to children regardless of income, potential for success, or cost of service. This legal responsibility prevents the "rationing" of resources. Not only would such rationing be illegal, it would also be highly unethical (Winterfield, 1995).

Client Population

Clients who come into the child welfare system do so involuntarily. "Clients do not usually come to the system looking for help, and once in the system, are often resistant, if not hostile, to the 'help' that is offered" (Feild, 1996, p. 5). Although clients are encouraged to actively participate in case planning and service provision, their freedom to terminate services often has serious negative consequences, including loss of contact with their families and ultimately termination of parental rights. Situations brought to the child welfare system also involve more than an individual client. The primary client is the child, but within the context of his or her family and the community. In fact, the client system most likely includes an array of people, their interactions with each other, and the full environment in which they live.

Span of Autonomy

Contrary to common belief, the child welfare agency does not have the ultimate power to decide the type and length of services to be provided for each child and family. The passage of PL 96–272 in 1980 mandated various case reviews under the direction of the court system. Final decisions regarding placements, reunification of families, and potential termination of parental rights are made in juvenile or family court by judges who may or may not agree with the recommendations of the child welfare caseworker. This oversight of child welfare practice and decisions regarding children and families by the court differs among jurisdictions across the country. Additionally, the court system has been financially and administratively unprepared for the mandated processes of "reasonable efforts" determination and ongoing reviews of child placement and family reunification. This has caused a substantial overload in the court system and a degree of tension between courts and the child welfare agencies. "Some judges estimate that 50% of their court time is allocated to the abuse and neglect calendar, which constitutes less than one-third of the total case filings" (Rubin, 1996, p. 47). In this climate, it is highly doubtful that the rationing of services, or denial of needed services due to capitation or other cost containment measures of managed care, will be taken into consideration by most judges when they are deciding which interventions are necessary for specific children and their families.

Treatment Protocol

Child welfare assessment and diagnostic practice skills are weak, and there is little ability to empirically link symptoms, diagnoses, interventions, and outcomes. For a number of reasons, evaluative data have been and continue to be lacking. Few child welfare agencies allocate funding to program or practice evaluation, and critically needed longitudinal studies are rarely undertaken. One exception to this lack of evaluation is the multitude of outcome studies on family preservation. Several efforts to determine the efficacy of family preservation services have produced mixed results and spurred intense debate on whether these services actually place children at risk of more harm. While there has been ample discussion of the limitations of the evaluative methodology used in these studies, a fairly clear picture of inconsistent application of a practice model has emerged.

Added to the fact that few child welfare agencies consistently apply an articulated model of practice, child welfare service delivery is plagued by a dearth of reliable, empirically based measurement tools. Unable to support the contention that the services being provided are actually working, child welfare continues to be viewed as ineffective, and its value is subject to speculation and harsh criticism. In an effort to fill this gap by developing empirically based outcome measures, the American Humane Association and American Public Welfare Association have cosponsored an annual series of roundtables bringing together child welfare researchers, administrators, and practitioners. Although the field is beginning to make progress in this area, much work is yet to be done.

Underlying managed care principles is the link between services provided and measurable outcomes. Child welfare must meet the challenge of defining outcomes for which the system actually has responsibility and that it can control if managed care is to have a chance of succeeding. Serious questions exist about the competency and ability of the child welfare system based on both unrealistic expectations and continued inadequate results, and a managed care system by its very nature could be viewed as placing children in danger. Constraints on removing children from risky situations, early reduction in levels of care, and premature family reunification may create a backlash against the managed care program and the child welfare system. Exceptional care should be taken in defining and crafting measurable outcomes (Feild, 1996).

Fiscal Constraints

Fiscal survival is the primary reason that physical and behavioral health care developed managed care systems and that its principles are now being brought to child welfare. Child welfare has historically been insufficiently funded, and all indications are that fiscal constraints will continue and possibly worsen. Child welfare agencies are experiencing budget deficits, and in many states substantial reductions of staff have resulted. The potential for containing child welfare costs and the possibility, even if remote, of actually cutting costs is seen as the major benefit of managed care in this era of fiscal accountability.

Feild (1996) identifies four factors that affect potential cost savings in child welfare: 1) high-cost placements, 2) underserved clients, 3) payment levels, and 4) intake and investigation protocols. Reducing high-cost placement through a managed care program will undoubtedly allow cost savings. For example, when several placements costing $5,000 per month are reduced to $3,500, substantive decreases in the cost of care are achieved. If fiscal incentives to reduce placement costs can be set at levels that do not offset cost savings, agencies will respond accordingly. In states or counties with large populations in high-cost placements, substantial savings are expected. In jurisdictions with few high-cost placements, however, savings will not be as dramatic and costs could actually increase as a result of fiscal incentive packages.

In many areas, few services are available to children and families. Under a managed care plan, an array of basic services is offered. For currently underserved areas, cost savings may not be realized. In fact, in such areas an increase of service provision may be necessary, and the cost of services may therefore rise. Conversely, some jurisdictions provide a rich array of services. In those areas, when services that have been provided are discontinued under the managed care plan, there could be cost savings, although they are likely to be quite small.

Private not-for-profit agencies are often not fully reimbursed for their actual service costs and rely on various funding mechanisms to cover their deficits. Under managed care these agencies could receive full or higher payments that would then result in no saving of public funds. Provider agencies must also be cautioned that with the potential increase in funding come expectations of measurable outcomes, stricter accountability, and service limitations.

A pivotal area for cost savings centers on the functions of intake and investigations. Children who eventually are placed in substitute care must first be identified as abused or neglected or at risk of maltreatment. The number of referrals received and determined appropriate for investigation will have a direct impact on the number of children and families served. If placement services are assigned to a managed care system but intake and investigative functions are retained solely by the public agency, the success of managed care could be jeopardized. Care must be taken to ensure that the protocols for intake and investigation complement the goals of managed care without violating the mandates of child protection and family preservation.

Although these unique characteristics of child welfare must be taken into consideration, they should not be viewed as unsurmountable obstacles to the implementation of managed care.

POTENTIAL BENEFITS OF MANAGED CARE

A number of child welfare practitioners see the movement into managed care as folly and warn of inevitable disaster. Others view the movement as an opportunity to make much needed substantive changes in a system that is floundering and may be facing its end.

Child welfare administrators, practitioners, and scholars are often the first to admit that the system needs overhaul. Just as accountability, cost savings and containment, and successful outcomes became a necessity in physical and behavioral health care services, so it is with child welfare. It is time for the child welfare field to take a progressive stance and consider viable options outside the mainstream child welfare service delivery system. Several areas, though challenging, provide opportunities to improve the delivery of services to children and families.

Assessment and Diagnostic Tools

Decision making in child welfare is often based on practice wisdom and the erratic use of poorly developed and untested assessment tools. Highly trained, experienced caseworkers confess to making decisions on "intuition." If a case presents a number of "red flags" or invokes a "gut feeling," a worker may determine that the child is at risk without empirical evidence to support the decision. Few of the risk assessment tools and family functioning scales typically used in decision making have been empirically tested, and even those that have are often used haphazardly and without adequate training. With appropriate and accurate standardized clinical tools to determine risk and target services, decision making would be consistent and defendable.

Feild (1966) cautions, however, that allowing a private managed care company to develop these protocols could result in restriction or denial of services to children and families deemed at risk by public child welfare. She recommends that public child welfare maintain control of the development of assessment and diagnostic tools to assure protection of the agency and its clientele. This is an area where collaboration between public child welfare and the managed care organization is needed. Given opportunity and guidance, tools to aid in systematic decision making can be developed by the professionals who will actually use them.

Systematic decision making is integral to the support of best practice standards. Currently, child welfare practice standards center on compliance with rules and regulations. Quality assurance reviews are for the most part examinations of case records to ascertain completion of required forms and other documentation. This type of review misses the essence of child welfare services and best practice standards. Quality assurance reviews based on actual services provided and their outcomes, as required under managed care, should provide information needed to substantiate success and identify areas in need of revision.

New Treatment Modalities

The problems faced by children and families brought to the attention of the child welfare system have not changed since its inception. Unfortunately, neither have most of the methods used to alleviate these problems. Given the overall poor results, we should not overlook the opportunity managed care may bring to develop new treatment methods. Obviously lacking in most child welfare agencies, both public and private, is an articulated, consistently used model of practice. More often than not, interventions are conducted with little or no attention to the theoretical foundation of a specific treatment modality. Services are provided without definitive planning based on the needs of the individual child and family. Although individual service plans are developed, they are often in boilerplate format and exclude any definitive treatment. Caseworkers regularly report intervening with children and families without thoughtful plans, often "flying by the seats of their pants" when making case decisions. With an identified model of practice, specific protocols would be followed based on accepted theoretical foundations, would use accepted and validated practices, and would be answerable to quality assurance reviews.

The flexibility of managed care funding can provide substantial opportunity to design and employ a variety of new intervention methods. In addition to improving mandated categorical services, of special interest is the opportunity to develop and implement prevention programs. Prevention programs are vital to managed care's success in cost containment. The potential in child welfare is all but unlimited.

Inherent in a managed care model is the evaluation of service delivery. Such evaluation makes it possible to determine what specific interventions are successful, with whom, and how they relate to specific outcomes. With the exception of family preservation, there has been little evaluation of child welfare services. Practice and program evaluation will provide the data necessary for ongoing planning, to substantiate outcomes, and to support requests for funding. Policymakers and the general public see the billions of dollars supporting the child welfare system as ill spent. They want success. Managed care may give child welfare the opportunities to develop the tools and interventions that help children and families achieve that success.

SUMMARY

The landscape of child welfare administration and practice is changing. Doty (1996) predicts:

> Some child welfare and child mental health provider organizations will sit back and watch as the volatile changes in the coming years play out. These will be the casualties. Other service providers will assume proactive leadership positions and participate in "inventing their own future." These will be the organizations that survive and thrive. All provider organizations, including both the "observers" and the "leaders" . . . , will experience dramatic, even fundamental change in the way they function and provide services. (p. 8)

The number of mergers and acquisitions among managed care service providers has been growing significantly. Child welfare has caught the eyes of those corporations constantly on the prowl for potential profits. This sets the scene for the possibility, if not the certainty, of a proprietary conglomerate of child welfare service providers. Should this be realized, public child welfare, the cornerstone and last bastion of primary host social work practice, will fall prey to the direction and control of management practices based on profit making and cost containment.

It must be remembered that "the provider serves as the gatekeeper, controlling access to services, controlling utilization of services" (Feild, 1996, p. 20). A critical element in the movement of child welfare into a managed care environment is the choice of designated service provider. Public and private child welfare agencies must work together to maintain their positions in service delivery and use this opportunity to redesign a system that meets its mandates, provides an array of services that result in successful outcomes, and is accountable to both its clients and societal constituents.

Redesign based on accountability and successful outcomes is long overdue in this professional field of practice. Although the ongoing problems within the child welfare system can be traced to the escalation of societal problems and cumulative inadequate funding, a portion of the responsibility must be assigned to the leaders of the field. The time has come to think and act for the future. By understanding the principles and elements of managed care and how they interact with the goals and characteristics of child welfare, it will be possible to move forward with caution and prudence. Sound strategic planning must be employed in the restructuring of the child welfare system, and managed care is one option under consideration. This great opportunity for child welfare must not be allowed to slip away.

REFERENCES

Allen, M. L. (1991). Crafting a federal legislative framework for child welfare reform. *American Journal of Orthopsychiatry, 61*(4), 610–623.

Authier, K. J. (1996). *Managed Care Update, 1*(1), 1–6.

Barth, R. P., Courtney, M., Duerr Berrick, J., & Alpert, V. (1994). *Pathways to permanence: Child welfare services pathways and placements.* Hawthorne, NY: Aldine de Gruyter.

Brodkin, E. Z., & Young, D. (1989). Making sense of privatization: What can we learn from economic and political analysis? In S. Kamerman & A. Kahn (Eds.). *Privatization and the welfare state.* Princeton, NJ: Princeton University Press.

Cohen, N. A. (Ed). (1992). *Child welfare: A multicultural focus.* Boston: Allyn and Bacon.

Courtney, M. E. (1995). The foster care crisis and welfare reform. *Public Welfare, 52,* 27–33, 40–41.

Doty, D. W. (1996). Managed care: What is it, where did it come from, and where is it going? *Managed Care Update, 1*(2), 1–8.

Emenhiser, D., Barker, R., & DeWoody, M. (1995). *Managed care: An agency guide to surviving and thriving.* Washington, DC: Child Welfare League of America.

Feild, T. (1996). *Managed care and child welfare: Are they compatible?* Bethesda, MD: Institute for Human Services Management.

Gil, D. (1981). The United States against vs. child abuse. In L. Pelton (Ed.), *The social context of child abuse and neglect.* New York: Human Science Press.

Goerge, R. M., Wulczyn, F. H., & Harden, A. W. (1995). *Foster care dynamics 1983–1993: An update from the multistate foster care archive.* Chicago: University of Chicago, Chapin Hall for Children.

Grubb, W. N., & Lazarson, M. (1982). *Broken promises: How Americans fail their children.* New York: Basic Books.

Halfon, N., English, A., Allen, M. L., & DeWoody, M. (1994). National health care reform, Medicaid, and children in foster care. *Child Welfare, 73,* 99–115.

Jimenez, M. A. (1990). Permanency planning and the Child Abuse Prevention Act: The paradox of child welfare policy. *Journal of Sociology and Social Welfare, 17*(3), 55–72.

Kempe, C. K. (1962). The battered child syndrome. *Journal of the American Medical Association, 181,* 17–34.

Lindsey, D. (1994). *The welfare of children.* New York: Oxford University Press.

Maas, H. S., & Engler, R. E., Jr. (1959). *Children in need of parents.* New York: Columbia University Press.

McCullough, C. (1996a). Developing a managed care approach to child welfare: Essential tools and critical investments. Washington, DC: Child Welfare League of America.

McCullough, C. (1996b). Managed care and child welfare: A Child Welfare League of America perspective. Washington, DC: Child Welfare League of America.

McCullough, C. (1996c). Survey on managed care and child welfare March 1996: The state of the states. Washington, DC: Child Welfare League of America.

McGowan, B. (1990). Family-based services and public policy: Context and implications. In J. Whittaker, J. Kinney, E. Tracy, & C. Booth (Eds.), *Reaching high-risk familes.* Hawthorne, NY: Aldine de Gruyter.

McGowan, B. (1990). Child welfare: The context for reform. In *Child welfare reform* (pp. 21–55). New York: Columbia University, National Center for Children in Poverty.

Mordock, J. B. (1996). The road to survival revisited: Organizational adaptation to the managed care environment. *Child Welfare, 75*(3), 195–218.

Morton, E. S. (1993). The evolution of family preservation. In E. S. Morton & R. K. Grigsby (Eds.), *Advancing family preservation practice.* Newbury Park, CA: Sage.

Pecora, P. J., Whittaker, J. K., & Maluccio, A. N. (1992). *The child welfare challenge.* New York: Aldine de Gruyter.

Rubin, H. T. (1996). The nature of the court today. *The Future of Children, 6*(3), 40–52.

Sarri, R., & Finn, J. (1992). Child welfare policy and practice: Rethinking the history of our certainties. *Children and Youth Services Review, 14*(3/4), 219–236.

Stein, T. J. (1991). *Child Welfare and the law.* New York: Longman.

Strausbaugh, J., & Drissel, A. (1997). Child welfare privatized: Kansas first state to try it. *Children's Voice, 6*(3), 27–29.

Tatara, T. (1994). The recent rise in the U.S. Child substitute care population: An analysis of national child substitute care flow data. In R. Barth, J. Duerr Berrick, & N. Gilbert (Eds.), *Child welfare research review.* New York: Columbia University Press.

U.S. Department of Health and Human Services, Administration for Children and Families. (1996). Child welfare, foster care, adoptions and Title IV-A. In *The green book* [unpublished update]. Washington, DC: Author.

U.S. Department of Health and Human Services, National Center on Child Abuse and Neglect. (1996). *Child maltreatment in 1994: Reports from states to the National Center on Child Abuse and Neglect.* Washington, DC: Author.

U.S. General Accounting Office. (1995). *Child welfare: Complex needs strain capacity to provide services* (GAO/HEHS Publication No. 95–208, Foster Care Overview). Washington, DC: Author.

Wexler, R. (1995). *Wounded innocents.* Buffalo, NY: Prometheus Books.

Winterfield, A. P. (1995). Managed care, privatization, and their impact on the child welfare system. *Protecting Children, 114*(4), 3–6.

Woodard, J. (1996, September). Funding systems: Defining federal programs. Paper presented at the Child Care Administrators Conference, Austin, TX.

CHAPTER 3

Current Practices in Public Child Welfare

John Mordock

Consultant; and former Assistant Executive Director,
Astor Home and Child Guidance Centers

Proponents of managed care argue that changes linked to capitated financing can help ameliorate three of the most dysfunctional aspects of the child welfare system. These include frequent foster care placements, long lengths of stay of those placed in foster care, especially those placed in group homes and congregate child care institutions, and the use of traditional family foster care in lieu of kinship foster homes.

This chapter focuses on the recent introduction of managed care practices in child welfare. Included in the discussion are aspects of managed care that are an extension of previous child welfare practices, as well as those new to child welfare. The discussion builds on and extends earlier discussions of the systematic changes needed by child welfare agencies in a managed care environment (Mordock, 1966b, in press). Some of these changes are the replacement of traditional purchase-of-service activities with capitated contracts; an array of services whose protocols are more standardized; interorganizational networks to create a seamless continuum of care, thereby diminishing fragmentation and gaps in community-based child welfare services; and data on service efficiency and effectiveness.

HISTORICAL BACKGROUND

In response to the large number of children who tended to languish in child care institutions and in other foster care settings, the Child Welfare Reform Act of 1979 was aimed at rescuing children from "foster care limbo" (Fanshel & Shinn, 1978). Regulations were passed that required foster care agencies to move children out of congregate care into community settings within two years of admission or to show cause in the local family court as to why they had not done so. Agencies were required to return children to their natural parents or free them for adoption. Permanent foster care for children was not an approved option. These activities were called permanency planning.

An impetus to develop community-based services was stimulated by the emergence of the permanency planning movement, one aspect of which was later called "family preservation" efforts (Adams, 1994; Maluccio, Fein, & Olmstead, 1986). This movement was assisted by passage of PL 96–272, the Adoption Assistance and Child Welfare Act of 1980, which created financial incentives to develop programs to prevent out-of-home placement and to reunify families. Funds were made available to combat the causes of child abuse or neglect and to link children and families with needed community services. In response, many child welfare agencies developed preventive services to help families with children at risk of placement; support services to foster parents were also developed, and child welfare agencies attempted to free children for adoption and provide adoption services.

While many young children in placement profited from the push for permanency planning and family preservation efforts, many emotionally disturbed children and adolescents in congregate care did not (Lerner, 1988). The original idea behind reducing time in congregate care facilities was that this could be done by making services available to youngsters in their home communities, but paralleling the deinstitutionalization movement in mental health, these services did not in fact become available. As a result, many youth were reinstitutionalized. With child welfare institutions having been closed and downsized, there was a consequent increase in admissions of youth to psychiatric hospitals (Weithorn, 1988), where services were brief and more circumscribed.

Escalating and persistent poverty, family violence, mental illness, and the drug epidemic have resulted in a substantial increase in foster care placements since 1985, and a corresponding increase in costs, in spite of permanency planning and family preservation efforts. In 1993, there were 2,898,000 child maltreatment reports, representing a twentyfold increase from 1963. Federal and state expenditures for child protection programs and associated foster care now exceed $6 billion a year (Coats, 1995).

By the end of 1993, 460,000 children were in foster care, up from 349,000 cases in 1988 and 276,000 cases in 1985 (Coats, 1996; U.S. Department of Health and Human Services, 1996). More than 659,000 children were served in the system during that year (Halfon, English, Allen, & DeWoody, 1994). At least another 100,000 are projected to be in the system by 1996. The cost of the federal share, both in maintenance payments and administrative training costs, grew from $891 million in 1988 to $2.7 billion in 1994, an increase of 300 percent (U.S. Department of Health and Human Services, 1996).

INTRODUCTION OF MANAGED CARE INTO CHILD WELFARE PRACTICE

In an effort to reverse the trend of increased foster care placements, managed care concepts are being introduced throughout the country. Managed care concepts stress that each child served will receive a level of care appropriate to the child's needs and will have an expedited permanency plan. Focus will be on reducing recidivism, preparing youth who are aging out of the system (becoming adults) with meaningful independent living skills, including job opportunities, and measuring client satisfaction with services (Child Welfare Administration [CWA], 1995).

It is anticipated that states and counties will develop and implement performance-based contracts (for example, only 30% of children served will be placed in foster care; 80% of children placed in foster care will be discharged within one year of placement) with child welfare providers who would be responsible for managing out-of-home care within a capitated fiscal structure. The hope of governmental agencies is that managed care will reverse the trend toward dramatically increased costs in foster care.

A number of child welfare agencies have been operating in systems that make them more ready for managed care practices than agencies that work in other systems. First, unlike mental health agencies, where funds came from purchase-of-service arrangements with payers, child welfare agencies have been subject to governmental rate-setting methodologies for many years. They always received fixed amounts to serve families in need. It can be argued that child welfare agencies are already managed, but they are not capitated.

Per diem rates for each child served are set by state social services departments based on a reimbursement formula. Initial rates were determined by examining the state's historical cost data from agencies that provided different types of foster care. Costs were subject to screens that set limits on spending in specific budget categories, such as administrative and operating costs. Rates are adjusted annually utilizing a set of factors including, but not limited to, a nondirect care cost parameter, a hold harmless percentage, a growth adjustment factor, and an annual inflation factor.

Funding through approved rates could be considered a form of quasi capitation, since agencies are not required to spend the per diem rates in predetermined ways on each child; they can, and do, spend more monies serving some children than others. Preventive services contracts, while negotiated to serve a fixed number of clients at any one time, also do not require that funds received are spent equally on all clients served.

Under managed care, it is intended that agencies will be given an up-front amount of money, capitated per child, calculated on historic rates multiplied by a predetermined number of anticipated care days. If the agency discharges a child before the child's care-day capitation level has been met, the agency can use the remaining funds for enhancing aftercare and other services. If the agency fails to reduce care days to expected levels, then the agency could lose money.

Under the older per diem system, where money flows for each day a child is in care, there are no fiscal incentives for agencies to decrease the lengths of stay for children in foster care. Proponents of managed care concepts believe that capitated funding systems will create fiscal incentives to develop service delivery systems that keep youth out of care, place children who need out-of-home in the least restrictive level of care, and reduce the lengths of stay of those in care. It is believed that fiscal incentives will encourage agencies to address the critical shortage of family foster homes, decrease the current use of high-cost congregate care, and subcontract with mental health agencies to rectify the present lack of adequate behavioral health care services for children and for the families of children in care.

Second, many child welfare agencies have developed considerable experience using different funding streams to support an array of services for children. Agencies use programs that divert children from foster care, even when these programs place stress on their foster care divisions. If the rate-setting system disappears from child welfare as it has in mental health, agencies with these experiences will fare better than agencies without these capabilities.

The overwhelming majority of hospitals and health systems throughout the United States negotiate payments with groups needing their services rather than receive state-established rates. Movements have begun that forecast this development in child welfare. Several counties in New York State have developed contracts with selected agencies that pay one rate for congregate care of eight months or less and a different rate of aftercare services lasting as long as four months. In other states, counties have issued requests for proposals calling for respondents to propose a rate for their proposed service arrangements.

Third, those agencies that are accredited by professional associations which require compliance with specified performance standards and that monitor compliance through the use of quality assessment and improvement practices will be better prepared for managed care than others.

While those agencies that are experienced in using per diem rates to serve children differently and in maintaining compliance with accrediting bodies should adapt readily to managed care practices, they, along with less sophisticated agencies, will need to develop some additional procedures to remain competitive in the managed care marketplace. These procedures include the definition of best practices, development of performance standards, procedures for immediate access to utilization information, procedures to actively involve clients in intervention planning, outcome assessment methods to determine cost-effectiveness, and formation of interagency networks. Each of these procedures will be discussed below.

Best Practices

A best practice is a state-of-the-art service or program that will optimize client outcomes at the least cost. Defining best practice has the following steps:

Identifying content of each service component

Describing how components fit together

Identifying the number of staff or staffing ratios required to deliver the service

Specifying staff credentials

Specifying consumer eligibility

Identifying the expected frequency of service sessions or the length of stay in the service

In child welfare, very little information exists about best practices. While the Homebuilders model (McKinney, Haapala, & Booth, 1991), promulgated nationwide as a model of intervention to prevent foster care placement (Adam, 1994), has articulated each of the five steps required of a best practice, others have replicated the model with different staff ratios, different eligibility criteria, and different outcomes.

In general, many child welfare practices are poorly defined and most services include a variety of different practices within the services offered. For example, in residential treatment settings there are educational, recreational, clinical, and social services, yet significant variation occurs among residential centers in staffing patterns, staff interactions with clients, program models, and lengths of stay. Another example is the existence of identical admission criteria to a variety of different group care settings..

Forsyth stated that prevention programs failed because the monies deployed were not specifically targeted at families of children at imminent risk of placement but were used instead to serve many needy families whose children did not meet this criterion (quoted in Lerner, 1988). In other words, these programs failed to apply the concept of "best practice."

Under managed care practices, providers will be expected to develop specific service protocols for clients with differing conditions. Each protocol must include the specific steps taken to achieve an objective. The steps must be clear to both the client and funding source. Such protocols both allow for uniformity in service delivery and contribute readily to the development of related outcome measures.

Terkelsen (1980) discusses assessing families in terms of three levels of goal attainability. The highest level is *full restoration*. At this level the family recaptures its capacity to promote the need attainment of all its members following each episode of service delivery in a community-based service center.

The second level is *supplementation*. Here the family is not expected to attain sufficiency in and of itself at any time. The service plan deliberately includes creation of some more or less permanent attachment between the family and an external helping agent. The family becomes semiautonomous. Involvement in self-help support groups or continual support by agency staff will always be required to preserve family stability.

The lowest level is *replacement*. Too much is missing in the family, so the family needs extensive supplementation to function adequately. One or more of its members will require continual involvement with a case manager, with many needing periodic placement in out-of-home settings. If capitated rates are set too low, the resources available will be inadequate to either supplement or replace high-risk families.

Performance Standards

In lieu of practice guidelines, child welfare agencies are increasingly expected to achieve specific performance standards set by funding sources. Some states have developed performance standards, sometimes referred to as general practice guidelines, to accompany the performance-based contracts awarded to provider agencies. For example, contract agencies in Ohio are expected to have written guidelines that include a statement that all children entering care or requiring protection must be served; no child can be excluded for reasons of retardation, developmental disability, mental illness, substance addiction, and so forth. These agencies are also expected to make available a full array of child welfare services and placement options. The initial placement of the child is determined by all involved parties. The child must be moved through the system of care based on identified goals and desired outcomes to the least restrictive setting. The agency, in conjunction with child protective services staff, determines when the child is to be moved out of care (Palmer, 1996).

Information Management Systems

A sophisticated information system is necessary in order to implement a capitated system. Considerable information is needed by child welfare agencies before they can calculate actual foster care costs, particularly congregate care costs for select groups, and set a valid capitated rate for the population they expect to serve. For example, the following data are required to determine the actual cost of serving certain categories of children in a specific population of children:

1. Percentages of cases admitted to foster care according to different placement types (such as persons in need of supervision, planned vs. emergency placements)
2. Percentage and total number of cases served per level of care (subsidized

adoption, kinship foster homes, family foster homes, therapeutic foster homes, group home care, institutional care, residential treatment)

3. Percentages and total number of cases according to different permanency planning goals (service needs of each group will differ)

4. Number of children needing community-based services and costs of these services

5. Monthly average number of beds and vacancies at different levels of care throughout the year

6. Average lengths of stay by different cohorts (such as age at admission, special needs, gender, permanency planning goals)

7. Percentages of first-time placements, planned placements, and emergency placements

8. Money spent under the capped Medicaid rate

9. Numbers and types of staff that can be assigned to the Medicaid rate

These data will enable an agency to know the actual cost of each service currently being provided to clients from a specific population, and to predict the cost of services if the continuum is used differently in the future. Initially, these data can be gathered manually. Eventually, however, an agency will need an information management system for rapid access to data.

Acquiring an information Management System.   Large agencies that plan to provide a full continuum of care themselves or to participate in a geographically dispersed partnership will need a comprehensive information management system (IMS). A seamless exchange of integrated information is required throughout the service network to help agencies determine the true costs of services rendered to specific populations of children.

The IMS should be compatible with existing agency systems and should allow agencies to identify, track, and chart variances between actual and expected services and outcomes; track and predict resource utilization by client population; document and monitor quality indicators and outcomes; generate problem lists for quick access to summaries of important client characteristics; access historical client data throughout the continuum of care; and provide graphical representation of trends and relationships.

Creating an Information Management System.   A considerable commitment in personnel, hardware, and software is required to implement a functional IMS. In spite of all the rhetoric about the need for electronic record keeping tied into an IMS (Corley, 1996), very few systems are operating in the United States. It can take over two years to get a system operational because there are always glitches, both following system installation and ongoing, in the system—the hardware, software, and telephone lines. Such systems require an administrator and paid staff to install and maintain the IMS and users at each site knowledgeable enough about the system to relate operational problems to IMS staff.

Client-Friendly Services and Client Satisfaction

Managed care principles include client-friendly services. Child welfare agencies are said to be client or family friendly when they value child and parent input, display a nonblaming attitude throughout their service delivery system, emphasize family strengths rather than deficits, and are readily available to meet both family-identified needs and respond to family requests.

New York City CWA's Project TOPP, for example, expects families served to select problem solutions and agencies to be guided by parent groups that help define service needs. Iowa's managed care program in child welfare outlines the involvement of families in service planning, policy making, and quality assurance (Nardini, 1996c).

Some fundamental differences in attitudes between agency staff and child protective services staff will cause initial difficulties in making managed care services family friendly. Family-friendly practices typically do not exist in child protective service-agencies, nor do its staff possess attitudes that nonprofit agency staff consider to be family friendly.

While one survey of child protective services clients revealed that some workers were viewed as helpful by clients (Magura, 1982), the experience by contract agency staff working in both prevention and foster care diversion programs suggests that most child protective services workers display an investigative attitude. They can resist joint service-planning efforts and expect contract agency staff to display the same investigative attitude and to explore issues of concern to child protective services (Nardini, 1966c). Their attitudes and expectations make it difficult for agency workers to develop the kind of open, emphatic interchange of information between worker and family that is needed to learn about the family's real needs and to develop consumer-driven service plans to meet these needs. Arriving at a consensus between child protective services staff, parents, and staff of contract agencies will not go smoothly in the initial stages of joint decision-making efforts (Nardini, 1996a, 1996b, 1996c).

To assess client satisfaction with services, child welfare agencies will need to survey clients, meet them in focused discussion groups, and establish client advisory boards. All surveys developed to assess satisfaction with specific services need to be user friendly and contribute to the evaluation of services provided and to outcome assessment.

Outcome Measurement

Some state departments of social services have generated requests for proposals calling for foster care prevention programs funded on a milestone-based approach. This perspective requires concrete outcomes for clients and specific performance targets as steps on the way to achievement of these outcomes. The outcomes are expected to be verifiable accomplishments, such as "90% of the children were absent from school for no more than 10 days during the school year," rather than small measurable pre-postdifferences. Outcome data also enable an agency to determine the costs associated with specific outcomes (Mordock, 1996a). The agency can answer such questions as, What is the actual cost for services necessary to reach various stages in the achievement of a permanency plan for an emotionally disturbed child with low intelligence?

Nonprofit child welfare agencies have used outcome data to improve their service delivery systems for some time (Astor Home for Children, 1963; Curry, 1991; Fahl & Morrissey, 1979; Fein, Maluccio, Hamilton, & Ward, 1983; Fein & Staff, 1993; McCroskey & Nelson, 1989; McMurtry & Gwat-Young, 1992; Milner, 1987; Mordock, 1978, 1988; Seaberg & Tolley, 1986; Weisman, 1994). Unfortunately, they have rarely discussed their findings in terms of the costs of achieving the outcomes observed.

In seeking to improve an outcome for some groups of children, some costs may actually need to increase while others can decrease. For example, in foster care prevention and diversion programs, service staff carry very small caseloads. Nevertheless, cost can be reduced by applying the service only to those most likely to benefit from the service.

Cost-Effectiveness

Managed care emphasizes payer-driven outcomes of cost containment and efficiency. The costs that need to be determined are the costs of achieving specified outcomes rather than the costs of providing services (Mordock, 1995).

For example, while the cost of therapeutic foster care for a child may be $45,000 per year, outcome data may reveal that only 50% of those served are successfully integrated into the community following discharge. Consequently, the actual cost of successful service is $90,000 per child because half the funds were wasted on children with unfavorable outcomes. Costs will be reduced only when the profile of the child most likely to profit from therapeutic foster care is identified and only when children with characteristics similar to or approaching this profile are admitted to therapeutic foster care.

While managed care proponents talk a lot about specific practice protocols, developing reliable and valid assessment instruments that will identify those most likely to profit from any circumscribed intervention takes considerable time and effort. In addition, moving from statistical probability, or children most likely to benefit, to a case-level decision, one about a specific child, becomes problematic. Unless the assessment instrument has an extraordinarily high confidence level, use of the decision rule will exclude some children from receiving an intervention who do not fit the profile but who would nonetheless benefit (false negatives) and will include those who fit the profile but who will not benefit (false positives).

Interagency Networks

Agencies preparing for managed care report making a number of changes in their organizations. While some of these are internal changes, the most significant changes are those related to involvement in networks.

It is unlikely that any child welfare agency can operate the full range of services needed by children at risk in a particular region. It is most likely that the full range of services will be offered by different agencies. Performance standards of funding sources will require that contract agencies have a no-rejection admission policy and a variety of different placement options available to serve each referred child in the least restrictive but most appropriate placement.

For example, in Massachusetts, eight private residential programs have entered into a partnership called the Child and Family Network of New England (Small, 1995). Plans call for member agencies to develop three centralized units, to centralize their intake, and to provide core services to each child and family admitted to any member agency. Figure 1 depicts the core services. Core services include assessment and short-term intervention, emergency shelter, respite, prevention and diversion services, nonresidential family programs, the full continuum of foster care, supervised apartment living, on-site technical services at schools, and health and mental health services.

The central management unit is designed to be the entity that formally contracts with social services and monitors client services. Children will be referred for placement to the central management unit. This unit will place each referred child in the member agency closest to the child's natural home that provides the needed level of care for the child. Each member agency has to either provide the core services itself or develop letters of agreement or subcontracts with community agencies to provide the services.

A second centralized unit is the family reunification, community, and educational inclusion services unit. This unit will remain involved with each family throughout its child's stay in care and during aftercare services, with the amount of involvement varying over the child's course of stay. Primary involvement would be to ensure the success of those children who are "stepping down" through the network. Unit staff would also troubleshoot cases and facilitate any necessary "time outs" from school, family, or residential placements. The reader is referred to Shulman and Athey (1993) for a description of how such a unit might be structured.

The third centralized unit is the training and research unit. Its purpose is to ensure that network standards are adhered to and that staff of member agencies are kept abreast of developments in the field.

FIGURE 1   Proposed Network Services

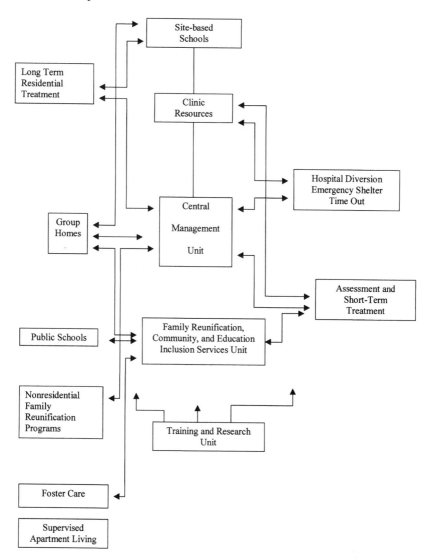

See Small (1995).

The leadership staff of the member agencies foresee a capitation scenario in which an agreed upon number of children would be served by their network for an annualized total dollar amount. (For example, the network would charge $10 million a year to serve 200 children, or $50,000 per child. This cost is roughly 10% less than the current annual cost for 200 children in congregate care.)

When considering forming a partnership, such as the one described above, some general principles should be followed. First, all members must understand clearly the real mission of each potential member. For example, some agencies may be looking for increased referrals rather than for ways to contribute to a fully integrated continuum of care. Others may be trying to dramatically decrease costs through the selective contracting process. Most health care networks that have formed throughout the United States, irrespective of the level of integration, have not shown increasing operating efficiency or an overwhelming ability to decrease costs (Ricks, 1996). The mere grouping of organizations does not, in and of itself, produce efficiency. The only reason for forming a partnership or network is the belief that the needs of children and families will be better met.

Second, small agencies that wish to be included in a network must offer very specialized services as well as be willing to contribute to the overall costs of the network infrastructure, such as the IMS, the ongoing quality assessment and improvement program, and the joint training of member agency staff. Members are needed that serve diverse and hard to treat populations, such as drug-addicted adolescents, violent adolescents, and the retarded disturbed, or that have very specialized units (for example, units for youth with chronic physical conditions, eating disorders, or severe learning disabilities).

Third, hospital departments of psychiatry, pediatric units of general hospitals, and medical multispecialty practices should be included in the network. Contracts with these physician groups can often be negotiated at lower rates if a higher volume of services is to be delivered. The partnership may consider leasing beds (also known as guaranteed beds) in psychiatric units because they can obtain discounted rates and promised access to a number of beds (Lazarus, 1996).

Fourth, credentialed clinicians must be used throughout the network to supervise the health and mental health services delivered in order to meet the requirements of accrediting bodies such as the National Committee for Quality Assurance and the Joint Commission of Healthcare Organizations (Dimmitt, 1995; "JCAHO vs. NCQA," 1996).

EXPERIMENTS IN MANAGED CARE

Before states adopt managed care practices on a large scale, policymakers will look at the result of demonstration projects that are taking place in various sections of the country. One such project, called Home Rebuilders

(HRB), began in 1993 and ended precipitously in 1995 after thirty months of operation. In this project, the New York State Department of Social Services and the New York City CWA agreed to capitate funding to six contracted agencies to serve a selected population of children. The agencies combined the expected per diem payments, kept at the 1993 level, over three years into a lump sum. It was estimated that the agencies would not lose money if their services resulted in a 10% care-day reduction for the targeted population over the three-year project.

In this model, the contract agencies made programmatic decisions independent from CWA. Excess pass-through monies were retained to reinvest in programs. Funds were moved from future years to the first year. Care days were rolled over from one year to the next. Cost savings were used to establish internal and external service delivery networks. Agency-developed IMSs were employed. There was freedom from programmatic review and oversight.

Both the outcomes observed and the money saved varied significantly among the six programs. For example, St. Christopher's–Jennie Clarkson placed its entire foster care population in the program (close to 800 children received project services over the thirty-month period; "Foster Care Model," 1995). The agency estimated 30% savings in year 3 and added these monies to the daily rate in years 1 and 2, giving it the enhanced, flexible funding needed to front-load services. While the project was directed primarily at reducing length of stay, the agency sought to significantly reduce recidivism by providing extended aftercare.

Services were defined at point of need, that is, the client's needs when problems began to develop. With the up-front money the agency hired a substance abuse counselor and five former clients as parent advocates to work closely with parents. Housing was a primary need for many clients. Classes were offered in child care, spiritual life, and the avoidance of domestic violence. There was a shift of influence from agency worker to parent. Parents could request a change in caseworker with no questions asked, and they could dictate the time and place of services. Intensive aftercare services were provided for nearly two years for some families rather than the ninety days of aftercare services required in traditional contracts. The agency's project director stated, "It is easy to design projects that get children out of care, but the greater challenge is to improve their quality of life in the community" (G. Kohomban, personal communication, September 19, 1965).

Over the project years, the permanency target was reported to have been exceeded by 14%, and length of stay was reduced by 17%. Thirty-seven percent of the foster children were returned home to their parents or adopted, compared to 28% of those in a randomly selected comparison group ("Foster Care Model," 1995). Of the 242 HRB children reunited with their families by project completion, only five reentered foster care, a recidivism rate of 2.07%. This is considerably lower than the prevailing New York City recidivism rate, which is reported to vary between 22% and 33%. Savings were $1.2 million in the first year and $840,000 in the second year. The agency planned to use these funds for extended aftercare, but the funding sources requested their return.

While HRB appears successful in reducing recidivism and returning children to the community (Courtney, 1995; Doyle, 1995; "Foster Care Model," 1995; McMahon & Cotter, 1996), several important variables were not controlled in the studies. Procedures for assigning children to treatment and control groups were unclear. Comparability of the two groups of children is uncertain. It is unclear how staff were selected to serve the two groups. Verbal reports indicate that in some agencies staff volunteered to serve the HRB group while in others supervisors selected staff to serve the group.

Regardless of the research shortcomings, these HRB projects created an opportunity to analyze managed care practices. Findings acquired from these HRB projects will be applied in today's more stringent fiscal climate, with significant differences expected between the HRB fiscal stream and the capitated model that states, counties, and cities will use in the future.

Based on a strong desire to implement capitated financing, the New York City CWA (1995) has developed a proposal for managed care, Project TOPP (Timely Outcomes–Permanent Placements), to be implemented in two phases. Under this model, service providers will assume full financial risk, with a safety net care-day reserve fund. The capitated rate is based on multiplication of projected care days and current per diem rate in phase I and on cohorts corresponding to particular characteristics of children in care of phase II. Funds may not be moved forward from later years, and deficits may not be rolled over from one year to the next; annual targets are specified by CWA; and procedural oversight is decreased in favor of a review of agency outcomes.

Nevertheless, a federal district court judge has issued a temporary restraining order against systemwide implementation of Project TOPP because of concerns that agencies might precipitously discharge some children. CWA has been required to submit to the court plans that describe in detail how children will be protected under the proposed funding system. If Project TOPP does get under way, more will be learned about implementation of managed care practices.

SOME PROBLEMS IN IMPLEMENTATION

Several problems must be addressed during implementation of a managed care system in child welfare. First, in some states, calculation of care rates will be complicated by the funding mechanisms of other systems that affect foster care. Increasing numbers of Medicaid-eligible children with special health care needs are being enrolled in managed health care programs. A study of expenditure data for children enrolled in the Maryland Medicaid program and in a private nonprofit health maintenance organization in Minnesota reported significant underpayment for high-risk children regardless of the capitation adjustment method. These data suggest that children with chronic health conditions would remain at risk for discrimination in a competitive health care market. As a result, the child welfare system would have to absorb the health care costs for children in foster care because a disproportionate number of foster care children experience chronic health conditions (Chernoff, Combs-Omre, Risley-Curtiss, & Heiserler, 1994).

Second, studies also reveal that between 29% and 48% of children in foster care show evidence of mental illness or emotional disturbance (Gries et al., 1995; Halfon, Mendonica, & Berkowitz, 1995; Pilowsky, 1995). Throughout the United States, foster care children have shown a disproportionately high utilization of mental health services (Chernoff et al., 1994; Frank, 1980; Halfon, Berkowitz, & Klee, 1992; Takayama, Bergman, & Connell, 1994).

In most states, children in foster care are ineligible for mental health care under managed care contracts. These children receive services at local mental health clinics. These clinics bill Medicaid for the services and supplement the inadequate Medicaid reimbursement with local and state funding. In New York, deficit funding has been replaced by an enhanced Medicaid system. Current plans call for this temporary reimbursement system to be replaced by funding allocated to state-approved provider networks to serve populations of seriously emotionally disturbed children, designated as special needs populations (SNIP), under a capitated funding system (Pataki, 1995). Currently, children in foster care in New York State will be excluded from services under these SNIP plans. Therefore, the future funding of mental health services for foster care children in New York State is uncertain.

Third, neither intensive case management nor a full continuum of mental health services necessarily reduces the need of children for out-of-home care (Bickman et al., 1994; Huz, Evans, Rahn, & McNulty, 1993). However, there is some evidence that these services can reduce the need for congregate care. Effective managed care practice requires the availability of a strong service system in the community. If the community lacks essential services, then such programs will be less effective. For example, in New York State 50% of the children who received intensive care management services had a mentally ill parent and 21% of those receiving preventive services to keep them out of foster care had a mentally ill parent (New York State Office of Mental Health, 1994). If the community lacks mental health services for these parents, more children will need out-of-home placements.

Fourth, in those communities rich in services, agency staff will spend considerable time and effort coordinating services for their clients. Interfacing with agencies providing services to a child or family requires considerable time. For example, in Iowa, clinical assessment and consultation teams, interagency teams established in five regions of the state, hold each month thirty-eight joint staffings and twenty-four case consultations (Nardini, 1996a). Such meeting time is costly and may not be practical in larger states.

Agency staff can encounter a variety of barriers in their efforts to coordinate services for clients. For example, a permanency plan for a child might require that a parent enroll in an outpatient substance abuse treatment center. Some centers have developed policies to reduce their waiting lists for services. For a child to be free for adoption, the agency must show diligent effort to rehabilitate the responsible parent. No family court judge would free a child for adoption simply because a parent missed a number of treatment sessions. Nevertheless, such delays can seriously hamper an agency's efforts to develop meaningful permanency plans for a child and can increase the child's length of stay care.

Finally, many families of high-risk youth have had extensive contact with social service and mental health agencies and have been labeled by these agencies as unmotivated and difficult cases. For example, if the mother misses a number of appointments, she may be unable to reapply for services for a specified time period, such as six months. Since disadvantaged clients, regardless of their pathology, regularly miss scheduled appointments (Mayer & Schamess, 1973; Mordock, 1996a), many clients can be denied treatment services for relatively long periods. Families can also perceive their child's problems as being exacerbated by professionals who overidentify with the child (Palmer, Harper, & Rivinus, 1983). Conversations with these families revealed that many felt that the agencies were unresponsive to their needs, inflexible in their approach, and uncoordinated, and that they emphasized an inadequate, individual-oriented approach to service delivery (Kaplan, 1986).

A WORD OF CAUTION

Proponents of managed care have stressed that intensive in-home services can divert most children from foster care and generate savings to be applied to new services. These predictions may be overly optimistic.

A number of studies suggest that relatively large numbers of children will continue to need foster care, and perhaps congregate care, during some portion of their lives. Adams (1994) summarizes the findings from recent independent evaluations of four foster home diversion programs and reports that intensive in-home services failed to make a significant impact on either the rate of foster home placements or the rate of congregate care placements.

Other studies have revealed that family preservation services are less effective with children from neglectful families (Bath & Haapala, 1993). Nearly twice as many children from such families were placed during service delivery than were children from abusive families. Youth who made the least progress in preservation programs presented complex histories of social problems including substance abuse, institutional placements, suicidal behavior, and running away, and they resided in homes where the mother was a victim of both domestic violence and sexual abuse (Werrbach, 1992).

Financial savings from capitated financing in the foster care system are unlikely to represent enough dollars to serve the countless numbers of families needing assistance. Redlener (1992) reports that between 500,000 and

700,000 children are homeless on any given night in the United States, and that at least eight million children are living in "housing endangered" conditions—conditions of profound squalor, transience, overcrowding, doubled- or tripled-up families—or with families considered profoundly "housing poor."

Some families will experience difficulty caring for children regardless of their economic conditions. Parents with profound mental illness, cognitive limitations, developmental disabilities, substance abuse problems, HIV infection, or physical health limitations will need assistance with child care. If their children are handicapped in some way, the need for assistance will be even greater. (The number of children with special needs adopted from foster care has increased by over 60% since 1993; U.S. Department of Health and Human Services, 1996).

However, there is some good news for managed child welfare. Parental willingness to participate in substance abuse services was highly predictive. Seventy-five percent of youth whose families refused recommended substance abuse services were placed during services. Children who avoid placement tend to be those with less delinquent behaviors and whose treatment plans specifically address the development of social supports (Spaid & Fraser, 1991).

CONCLUSION

While managed care is a term recently introduced to denote a policy change in child welfare practice, many practices subsumed under the term have been employed for some time. With a fixed amount of funds each year, child welfare agencies have allocated funds differentially to provide different services to children with different needs. Those agencies with a history of success in delivering diversified services to children and families can be expected to adapt successfully to managed care practices.

Even more sophisticated agencies, however, will need to develop practice guidelines and specific service protocols, implement an information management system to help staff determine service and outcome costs for different client groups, develop a provider network that will enable clients to receive a continuum of care, and collaborate with agencies that have different missions.

While the primary goal of managed care in child welfare is the prevention of out-of-home placement, data indicate that wholesale adoption of this outcome is unwarranted. Capitated rates need to be set with the knowledge that a significant number of families are not capable of full restoration. While the Home Rebuilders project suggests that generous capitated funding can promote community care of many high-risk children at lower costs, such funding will not prevent the need for foster care by a large number of children. Institutional and group care provides for all of a child's needs in one setting. The ability to replicate this network of services in all communities cannot be assumed. If a capitated rate is set too low, quality of services will be compromised and managed care will be just another term meaning limited resources to families in need.

REFERENCES

Adams, P. (1994). Marketing social change: The case of family preservation. *Children and Youth Services Review, 16,* 417–432.

Astor Home for Children. (1963). *What we have learned: A report on the first ten years of the Astor Home, a residential treatment center for emotionally disturbed children.* Rhinebeck, NY: Author.

Bath, H.I., & Haapala, D. A. (1993). Intensive family preservation services with abused and neglected children: An example of group differences. *Child Abuse and Neglect, 17,* 213–226.

Bickman, L., Guthrie, P. R., Foster, E. M., Lambert, E. W., Summerfelt, W. T., Breda, C. S., & Heflinger, C. A. (1994). *Final report of the outcome and cost/utilization studies for the Fort Bragg Evaluation Project (Vol. 1).* Nashville, TN: Vanderbilt Institute Center for Mental Health Policy.

Chernoff, R., Combs-Omre, T., Risley-Curtiss, C., & Heiserler, A. (1994). Assessing the health of children entering foster care. *Pediatrics, 93,* 594–601.

Child Welfare Administration. (1995). *A proposal for managed care: Project TOPP.* New York: City of New York Human Resources Administration, Child Welfare Administration.

Coats, D. (1995, July 13). Statements on introduced bills and joint resolutions. *Congressional Record* (Daily Ed.), *141,* S8255–S8265.

Coats, D. (1996, July 18). Personal responsibility, work opportunity, and Medicaid Restructuring Act of 1996. *Congressional Record* (Daily Ed.), *142,* S8105–S8150.

Corley, P. (1996, March/April). Putting the "managed" in managed care. *InfoCare,* p. 48.

Courtney, J. (1995). *Home Rebuilders at Little Flower: The second year.* Brooklyn, NY: Little Flower Children's Services.

Curry, J. F. (1991). Outcome research on residential treatment: Implications and suggested directions. *American Journal of Orthopsychiatry, 61,* 348–357.

Dimmitt, B. S. (1995, December). Accreditation: What's the big deal? *Business and Health,* 38–43.

Doyle, L. (1995). *Bronx Community Services Home Rebuilders report for fiscal year 7-1-94 to 6-30-95.* Bronx, NY: New York Foundling Bronx Community Services.

Fahl, M. A., & Morrissey, D. (1979). The Mendota model: Home community treatment. In S. Maybanks & M. Bryce (Eds.), *Home based services for children and families: Policy, practice, and research.* Springfield, IL: Thomas.

Fanshel, D., & Shinn, E. B. (1978). *Children in foster care: A longitudinal investigation.* New York: Columbia University Press.

Fein, E., Maluccio, A. N., Hamilton, V. J., & Ward, D. E. (1983). After foster care: Outcomes of permanency planning for children. *Child Welfare, 62,* 485–558.

Fein, E., & Staff, I. (1993). Last best chance: Findings from a reunification program. *Child Welfare, 72,* 25–40.

Foster care model attracts New York—but only in part. (1995, November 20). *The New York Times,* pp. A1, B4.

Frank, G. (1980). Treatment needs of children in foster care. *American Journal of Orthopsychiatry, 50,* 256–263.

Gries., L. T., Fribourg, A., Goldberg, F. H., Gonzales, M., Schneiderman, M., & Shaw, J. (1995). *Issues concerning the identification of children and adolescents eligible for special needs plans.* Committee on Psychologists of Voluntary Child Care Agencies, Sub-Committee on Special Needs Plan Criteria (available at 575 Lexington Avenue, New York).

Halfon, N., Berkowitz, G., & Klee, L. (1992). Mental health services utilization by children in foster care in California. *Pediatrics, 93,* 594–601.

Halfon, N., English, A., Allen, M., & DeWoody, M. (1994). National health care reform, Medicaid and children in foster care. *Child Welfare, 73,* 99–115.

Halfon, N., Mendonica, A., & Berkowitz, G. (1995). Health status of children in foster care: The experience at the center for the vulnerable child. *Archives of Pediatric Adolescent Medicine, 149,* 386–392.

Hux, S., Evans, M. E., Rahns, D. S., & McNulty, T. L. (1993). *Evaluation of intensive case management for children and youth: Third year final report.* Albany, NY: New York State Office of Mental Health, Bureau of Evaluation and Services Research.

JCAHO vs. NCQA: Battling for MCO accreditation. (1996, July/August). *InfoCare,* p. 14.

Kaplan, L., (1986). *Working with multi-problem families.* Lexington, MA: Heath.

Lazarus, A. (1996, April). Leased psychiatric beds. *Psychiatric Services, 47,* 351–352.

Lerner, S. (1988). *State-raised: Kids no one wants.* New York: Foundation for Child Development.

Magura, S. (1982). Clients view outcomes of child protection services. *Social Casework: The Journal of Contemporary Social Work, 63,* 522–531.

Maluccio, A. N., Fein, E., & Olmstead, K. A. (1986). *Permanency planning for children: Concepts and methods.* New York and London: Tavistock.

Mayer, H., & Schamess, G. (1973). The importance of maintaining long-term treatment services for the economically deprived family. *Psychosocial Process, 2,* 128–143.

McCroskey, J., & Nelson, J. (1989). Practice-based research in family support: The Family Connection Project example. *Child Welfare, 68,* 573–588.

McKiney, J. M., Haapala, D., & Booth, C. (1991). *Keeping families together: The Homebuilders model.* New York: Aldine de Gruyter.

McMahon, R. J., & Cotter, M. J. (1996). *Foster care and managed care: The Home Rebuilders program at St. Christopher–Ottilie.* Unpublished manuscript, St. Christopher–Ottilie Services for Children and Families, Sea Cliff, Long Island.

McMurtry, S. L., & Gwat-Young, L. (1992). Differential exit rates of minority children in foster care. *Social Work Research and Abstracts, 28,* 42–48.

Milner, J. L. (1987). An ecological perspective on duration of foster care. *Child Welfare, 66*, 113–123.

Mordock, J. B., (1978). *Ego impaired children grow up: Post discharge adjustment of children in residential treatment.* Rhinebeck, NY: Astor Home for Children.

Mordock, J. B. (1988). Evaluating treatment effectiveness. In C. H. Schaefer & A. J. Swanson (Eds.), *Children in residential care: Critical issues in treatment* (pp. 219–250). New York: Van Nostrand Reinhold.

Mordock, J. (1995). Program evaluation versus applied research: Performance targets, outcomes and user-based factors in evaluating children's treatment programs. *Residential Treatment of Children and Youth, 13*(2), 1–14.

Mordock, J. B. (1996a). The real world of the child guidance clinic. *Administration and Policy in Mental Health, 23*, 211–230.

Mordock, J. B. (1996b). The road to survival revisited: Organizational adaptation to the managed care environment. *Child Welfare, 75*, 195–218.

Mordock, J. B. (In press). Preparing for managed care in residential treatment. *Residential Treatment of Children and Youth.*

Nardini, C. W. (1996a, June). *Managed behavioral healthcare and the child welfare system in Iowa.* Paper presented at the Training Institute on Developing Local Systems of Care in a Managed Care Environment, Traverse City, MI.

Nardina, C. W. (1996b, August). *Managed behavioral healthcare and the child welfare system in Iowa.* Discussion with staff of the Central and Regional Offices of the Administration for Children and Families, Washington, DC.

Nardini, C. W. (1996c, September). *Managed behavioral healthcare and the child welfare system in Iowa.* Paper presented at a conference sponsored by the Office Administration for Children and Families, Seattle, Washington.

New York State Office of Mental Health. (1994, May). Parenting with mental illness. *OMH News, 6*(3).

Palmer, A. J., Harper, G., & Rivinus, T. M. (1983). The "adoption process" in the inpatient treatment of children and adolescents. *Journal of the American Academy of Child Psychiatry, 22*, 286–293.

Palmer, I. R. (1996, August). Managed care in child protection: Envisioning a new system for new realities. *Behavioral Healthcare, 5, 2, 4, 7.*

Pataki, G. (1995, March). *The Partnership Plan: Public-private initiative ensuring health care for needy New Yorkers.* Albany: State of New York.

Pilowsky, D. (1995). Psychopathology among children placed in family foster are. *Pediatric Services, 46*, 906–910.

Redlener, I. (1992, June 29). *Issues in Medicaid managed care.* Hearing before U.S. House Committee on Energy and Commerce. Washington, DC: Government Printing Office.

Ricks, C. S. (1996, March 25). Managed care will end era of provider networks. *Modern Healthcare*, p. 82.

Ryder, M. G., Courtney, J., & Ellis, B. (1994). *Home Rebuilders: The first year's experience at Little Flower Children's Services.* Brooklyn, NY: Little Flower Children's Services.

Seaberg, J. R., & Tolley, E. S. (1986). Predictors of the length of stay in foster care. *Social Work Research and Abstracts, 22*, 11–17.

Shulman, D. A., & Athey, M. (1993). Youth emergency services: A total community effort, a multi-system approach. *Child Welfare, 72*, 171–179.

Small, R. (1995, October). *Networks, mergers and managed care: The realities of agency change.* Paper presented at the annual conference of the New York Coalition of Children's Mental Health Services, Ellenville, NY.

Spaid, W. M., & Fraser, M. (1991). The correlates of success/failure in brief and intensive family treatment: Implications for family preservation services. *Children and Youth Services Review, 13*, 77–100.

Takayama, J., Bergman, A., & Connell, F. (1994). Children in foster care in the state of Washington. *Journal of the American Medical Association, 217*, 1850–1855.

Terkelsoen, K. G. (1980). Toward a theory of the family life cycle. In E. A. Carter & M. McGoldrick (Eds.), *The family life cycle: A framework for family therapy* (pp. 21–52). New York: Gardner.

U.S. Department of Health and Human Services (1996, June 11). *HHS invests in America's children* [press release].

Weisman, M. (1994, July). When parents are not in the best interests of the child: "family preservation" has become child-welfare dogma—but some children need institutional care. *Atlantic Monthly*, pp. 43–44, 46–47, 50–54, 56–60, 62–63.

Weithorn, L. (1988). Mental hospitalization of troublesome youth: An analysis of skyrocketing admission rates. *Stanford Law Review, 40*, 663–738.

Werrback, G. B. (1992). A study of home-based services for families of adolescents. *Child and Adolescent Social Work Journal, 9*, 505–523.

CHAPTER 4

System Reform in Public Mental Health: The Massachusetts Experience

Christopher G. Hudson

Professor, School of Social Work, and Executive Director,
Center for Applied Research and Development, Salem State College

The introduction of managed care in the public mental health system in Massachusetts has to date replicated the experience of earlier waves of policy innovation. Initial enthusiasm on the part of implementers has given way to the imperatives of political and economic accommodation, solving some problems but creating further fragmentation. This is not unexpected. Managed care is a broad term encompassing such diverse goals as cost containment and quality improvement, which, its proponents believe, can be achieved through an active managerial approach using techniques such as case management, preauthorization, utilization review, creation of provider circles, capitation, and performance contracting.

The story of managed care in Massachusetts is an unfinished one. In 1996 the state began implementing a second-generation, carved-out program for all Medicaid-funded services through a statewide behavioral health corporation. The first-generation implementation of managed care occurred between 1992 and 1996 and involved the establishment of a privately operated statewide mental health carve-out program. The current rendition of the program not only preserves this design but also dramatically expands its scope. It is intended to improve coordination between service systems by clearly differentiating the state mental health authority's continuing care program from the Medicaid-funded program for acute care. Before examining the specific experience since the 1992 introduction of behavioral health carve-out programs in the Commonwealth, this chapter will first review the major institutions and trends in the state that have combined to drive efforts to contain costs, privatize, and manage service delivery during the late 1980s and 1990s.

BACKGROUND

This section will discuss trends that predate and contribute to the managed care initiatives in the Commonwealth. It will then consider the role of managed care in the mental health policy development efforts of both the Dukakis (D) and Weld (R) administrations, which preceded and accompanied the introduction of the current carve-out programs in the Commonwealth.

Key Trends

The dramatic expansion of health care costs in the past twenty years has created considerable pressures for cost containment. Earlier efforts to contain costs, such as through the use of diagnosis-related groups, which were introduced into Medicare in 1982, focused on physical heath but exempted psychiatric services. For this reason, private psychiatric services had been one of the few growth areas in health care during the 1970s and early 1980s. It was an expansion that in part reflected efforts of providers to capitalize on the lack of controls and the traditional fee-for-service plans that were dominant in the mental health field (Dorwart & Epstein, 1993). It was not until the middle and late 1980s that health care purchasers began to control private psychiatric hospitalization levels.

The growth of private psychiatric inpatient services has contributed to the myth that the deinstitutionalization of mental hospitals had subsided by 1980. This view also arose from an official policy of many state mental health authorities to place a moratorium on the reduction of state hospital censuses as well as from official National Institutes of Mental Health statistics, which showed only a slight reduction in hospitalization levels between 1980 and 1990. These statistics reflected the inclusion of residential services into the same category as inpatient hospital services in NIMH statistical monographs and largely camouflaged the dramatic reductions in overall hospitalization levels during this period. According to the 1980 and 1990 U.S. Censuses, the total count of persons in all types of mental health inpatient units dropped by about one-half (52.7%) during the 1980s (see Hudson, Flory, & Friedrich, 1995, p. 11). Much of this drop was due to the decline in private psychiatric hospitalization in the later part of the 1980s, which was achieved mainly through shortened lengths of stay. For example, the Xerox Corporation has reported that the average length of stay of its employees in mental health facilities dropped from 33.7 days in 1987 to 9.9 days in 1994 (Iglehart, 1996, p. 133).

Probably the most important effect on this trend was the doubling of vacancy rates in private psychiatric hospitals in Massachusetts, from 10.5% in 1983 to 20.9% in 1988 (Manderscheid & Sonnenschein, 1990, p. 88). The growing vacancy rates contributed to a newfound interest on the part of private hospitals in negotiating arrangements with state officials to assume the care of those patients formerly seen as public wards. Thus, without the newest, but least visible, wave of deinstitutionalization, state administrators would have had little success in efforts to privatize and shift the costs of the seriously mentally ill to nonstate sources.

By the late 1980s, managed care and behavioral health companies had largely exhausted the corporate market and were looking to the public sector, in particular Medicare and Medicaid, as the next frontier (Essock & Goldman, 1995). The mental health components of these two federal programs had been, until the 1980s, dominated by institutional care (Manderscheid & Sonnenschein, 1990). The Reagan administration, however, had introduced the possibility of state waivers of selected sections of Titles XIII and XIX of the Social Security Act for the purpose of increasing state experimentation and permitting broader community services.

A relaxation of federal waiver requirements under the Clinton administration also made it possible for states to shift some of the costs of inpatient services to the federal government. Medicaid cannot be collected by certain institutions classified by the Health Care Financing Administration (HCFA) as "institutes of mental disorders"; this designation covers private and state mental hospitals 50% of whose clientele aged 18–65 have a primary diagnosis of mental illness. General hospitals with psychiatric units, however, are not affected by this regulation, nor are public health facilities with a minority of psychiatric patients. State officials have become increasingly sophisticated at circumventing the institute of mental disorder limitation, for example, through wraparound arrangements in which a general hospital manages and thereby wraps its license(s) around a state psychiatric unit. Such strategies directly serve local interests of cost containment, in particular cost shifting, because they transfer 50% or more of the costs of psychiatric care to the federal government through increased access to Medicaid payments.

Deinstitutionalization, as well as the imperatives of cost containment and cost shifting, has fueled the emergence of managed care companies in the public sector. As deinstitutionalization and privatization have developed in tandem (Hudson, Salloway, & Vissing, 1992), managed care has been the most recent facet of this megatrend to emerge. The introduction of behavioral health companies in public mental health privatizes not so much service delivery as the oversight of the service system. The impact of this shift is yet to be determined.

An examination of accompanying trends reflected in the Massachusetts experience provides only limited reasons for optimism. These include not only the accelerated shift from institutional to community care but also a shift from tertiary to secondary and preventive services. Agency and group-based practices are favored over private practice, short-term over long-term treatment, just as group and family modalities are being promoted over individual modalities. At the same time, a possible loss of autonomy and fragmentation of clinical decision making may offset whatever benefits could emerge from the other trends cited, especially if fiscal incentives are permitted to dominate professional decision making.

Dukakis Administration

During the 1980s state mental health was largely driven by the pressing need to redress the consequences of deinstitutionalization. These included the neglect of the seriously mentally ill and the fragmentation of the public mental health system in each state. In Massachusetts, as in many states, this meant narrowing the focus of the Department of Mental Health to the deinstitutionalized population through not only provision of case management but supported housing, clubhouses, and psychosocial rehabilitation. Massachusetts state officials carefully balanced their response to a powerful mental patients' rights movement led by Empower, and allied themselves with the burgeoning family movement, led by the Alliance for the Mentally Ill, which advocated both biological and rehabilitative services. In 1985 Governor Michael Dukakis released his special message, which committed the state to a dramatic expansion of community mental health services while maintaining a moratorium on reductions at its nine state hospitals with approximately 2,200 patients (Massachusetts Department of Mental Health, 1985).

The 1980s also included a period of protracted struggle between state mental health authorities and the former, federally funded community mental health centers. As the state mental health authorities became stronger through Reagan-era federal block grants, as well as through their alliance with patient and family groups, they sought to more actively manage their contracts with local mental health centers, typically by instituting some version of performance contracting or through a state case management system.

Despite the many ways in which the Department of Mental Health under the Dukakis administration sought to assume active control of its system of vendors, the rhetoric of managed care was not yet part of the program. Brotman (1992) points out that Massachusetts already had a de facto managed care system because its payments to its vendors were effectively capitated through the budgeting and purchase-of-service systems. In addition, it officially instituted in 1987 its "expanded brokerage" model of case management, in part to fulfill the requirements of the newly enacted federal Mental Health Planning Act of 1987. By 1992 the state would be providing case management services to 7,265 adults and 745 children (Leadholm & Kerzner, 1995, p. 549). However, it was only three years after Dukakis's 1985 special message that the recession made its effects felt. By 1988 staff freezes effectively aborted the ambitious five-year program outlined in that message.

The Dukakis administration set the stage for managed care through its attempts to control and manage its extensive and fairly autonomous system of vendors. Its rhetoric was one of public-private partnership rather than the "managed competition" and aggressive privatization of both services and administrative oversight functions that characterized the succeeding administration of Governor Weld. The Dukakis administration's targeting of the seriously mentally ill thus set the stage for a later policy shift back to less intensive, short-term services for those less disabled. This shift has been embodied mostly by the transition in Medicaid mental health services from institutional to community services under the managed care programs of the Weld administration.

Weld's "Reinvesting Government"

At the time William Weld was elected governor in 1991 the Commonwealth was in the midst of its worst, most unusually protracted recession in a decade. The state was in fiscal crisis. Taxpayers saw state government as bloated, inefficient, and expansive. The private sector was continuing to lose jobs (Leadholm & Kerzner, 1995, p. 543). Dramatic expansions in the Medicaid budget also contributed to this crisis.

As a moderate Republican, governor Weld had vowed to streamline and cut waste in government, to maintain and improve services while cutting costs through both reorganization and privatization. Reorganization in the mental health field was initially pursued through the appointment of a Special Commission on Hospital Consolidation. Its mandate was to streamline the state hospital system and to extend the principles of the Brewester consent decree. This decree, which had earlier established model community mental health services in the western part of the state, was to be extended through the rest of Massachusetts (Wisor, 1993). Privatization was also pursued through the successful application of HCFA for a waiver of 1915b regulations of the Social Security Act. This involved securing permission to establish the MassHealth Medicaid program, part of which involved subcontracting the management of all mental health and substance benefits under Medicaid to a private behavioral health corporation.

The interlocking trends of cost containment, deinstitutionalization, and privatization have driven the introduction of managed care in the public health arena in Massachusetts. Similarly, the rhetoric of private-public partnership under the Dukakis administration set the stage for a reluctant shift to the concept of managed competition under the succeeding Weld administration, a topic to which we will now turn.

DEPARTMENT OF MENTAL HEALTH INITIATIVES

Shortly after his election in 1991, Governor Weld appointed Eileen Elias, a veteran Department of Health employee, as the department's commissioner. By this time budget cuts had crippled the community mental health initiatives of the former administration. The challenge for the new Mental

Health administration was to find some way to "join its mission" with that of the new governor's, to design a cost-efficient system and, at the same time, continue its previous program development efforts (Leadholm & Kerzner, 1995). The new commissioner's strategy relied on a "comprehensive community service system/public managed care" (CCSS) initiative. This program had several components, which included closure or consolidation of several state hospitals as recommended by the special commission; reinvestment of saved resources in community care initiatives; reduction of area and site offices; introduction of an extensive participatory planning process; and cooperation with the Department of Public Welfare in its 1915b waiver program involving the establishment of the Medicaid-funded Massachusetts Mental Health Substance Abuse Program.

Beginning with the above changes, the department began embracing the rhetoric of public managed care:

> As a first step towards the development of public managed care, the Department has undertaken three major initiatives—the privatization of acute psychiatric inpatient services; the closure/consolidation of four of its state hospitals; and the movement of state hospitals funds to expand the community-based service system. These are three basic tenets of the development of public managed care. The term public managed care refers to a network of integrated comprehensive, accessible, quality, and flexible community based services. (DMH, 1993, p. 5)

Another department official attempted to define the department's public managed care policy as consisting of the implementation of a dozen key tenets, including 1) the centrality of privatization of service delivery; 2) the CCSS participatory planning process; 3) flexibility services characterized by continuity of care; 4) a case management system; 5) clinical services provided in the least restrictive environment; 6) quality management; 7) accountability and the defined expectations for the Department of Mental Health; and 8) targeted services for homeless and multicultural and linguistic minorities (Leadholm & Kerzner, 1995, p. 546). Although these tenets, as well as the preceding definition, outline several of the generic principles of mental health programming, only a few of them are commonly associated with managed care, most notably quality management. None specifically defines a managed care strategy as it is commonly recognized. By embracing some of the rhetoric of managed care, yet stopping short of implementing its most essential features, such as capitation, the department found itself having to follow the lead of the state Medicaid program in the development of a full-fledged mental health managed care program.

At the heart of the department's change efforts was the closure of state hospitals. Several of the hospitals, archaic and very costly structures built in the nineteenth century, were only being partially used, often for patients who were awaiting community placement or who had complicated dual diagnoses involving medical conditions, substance abuse, or development disabilities in addition to their mental illnesses.

On February 26, 1991, Governor Weld signed Executive Order 301, which established the Governor's Special Commission on Consolidation of Health and Human Services Institutional Facilities. After a rushed study of the feasibility of closures, the commission made recommendations on specific institutions.

On June 19, 1991, the commission submitted its recommendations to the governor for approval, and they were implemented shortly thereafter (DMH, 1993, p. 2). Mental health staff immediately undertook an extensive planning process for the closures, which were to be accomplished under tight time schedules and budgets. Metropolitan State Hospital was the first to be closed (January 1992), followed by Danvers State (June 1992) and Gaeblers Children Center (September 1992). In May 1993 the process was completed with the closure of Northampton State Hospital. The closures represented a reduction in patient census from 1,852 to 1,084 or 41.5%, over a two-year period. During this same time, 1,706 staff positions were eliminated. Between FY 1990 and FY 1994, $62 million was saved (DMH, 1993).

Most of the savings in the hospital system were achieved through privatization and cost shifting. The "closure" of Danvers State Hospital was something of a misnomer. The majority of the hospital's intermediate and long-term units were immediately reopened, with many of the same staff, at Tewksbury Hospital, a state public health facility that served mostly indigent older adults with long-term medical problems and that had considerable unused space. Despite the extensive costs for remodeling, this initiative saved the Department of Mental Health money by effectively transferring approximately one-half the Danvers State Hospital costs to the federal government. Tewksbury Hospital was not classified by HCFA as an institute of mental disorder and thus was eligible for Medicaid reimbursement for mental health services to adults between ages 18 and 65.

The admissions and short-term units from Danvers and other hospitals were relocated in private general hospitals with psychiatric programs. This move was accomplished through a contracting process in which the department agreed to be payer of last resort, after all possible payments were collected from third-party insurance sources such as Medicaid. In total, a dozen such short-term units were established throughout the state. This strategy would not have been possible if vacancy rates in such hospitals had not been particularly low. Furthermore, the department had recently been exempted from Public Health's determination-of-need standards, which tended to restrict the establishment of new medical units (Leadholm & Kerzner, 1995). Nonetheless, considerable planning and expenditures were required to assure that the new facilities would be reimbursable because Medicaid reimbursement requires that the facilities be HCFA certified and accredited by the Joint Commission for the Accreditation of Healthcare Organizations.

A key point of controversy between advocates and department officials was whether the costs of the new units would be greater or less than the expected savings. Most advocates eventually accepted the department's accounting, which showed $133.7 million in gross savings: $62 million from closures, $17.9 million from revenue enhancement, $11.1 million from staff insurance savings, and $42.7 million from saved renovation costs. In contrast, costs totaled $65.8 million: $26.7 million for inpatient replacement beds, $34.1 million for residential expansion, and $5 million for the placement of mentally retarded individuals. In total, net savings of $67.9 million could be claimed (DMH, 1993, p. 4).

The other development that contributed to the entry of privatization and managed care into inpatient care was the expansion of the community care system. At the center of this expansion was an extensive participatory planning process conducted in 1991 in each of the department's catchment areas. In the northeast area (northeast suburbs of Boston and Merrimack Valley areas), for instance, fifty to one hundred consumers, family members, and agency personnel took part in a half-dozen committees over a six-month period to assess needs and recommend new services. Although this was designed to be a "consumer-driven" system, the CCSS committees were frequently dominated by professionals who represented agency interests. Despite minimal systematic planning, these groups produced recommendations that highlighted particular areas of need, such as respite beds and programs for the dually diagnosed. The effort of these groups were supplemented by a statewide needs assessment contracted to the Human Services Research Institute, which relied on focus groups of consumers and professionals.

While the CCSS committees were generating their recommendations, department personnel were busy planning for a major expansion of the residential care system using monies saved from the hospital consolidation. This plan involved the addition of low-intensity residential beds, which permitted additional patients in moderate- and high-intensity homes to be transferred, thereby opening bed space for the more seriously disabled patients who were awaiting placement out of the state hospitals. A total of 625 new community residential beds were created between 1991–1992, and overall, 1,400 beds were added between 1990 and 1995. These new beds effectively transferred several hundred patients to the care of private vendor corporations, thereby creating a de facto managed care system operated through the department's purchase-of-service and case management systems.

At the same time that the community care system saw some expansion, such as emergency services, respite beds, and clubhouses, traditional community mental health centers had to increasingly restrict psychotherapeutic services to those with third-party coverage. Those centers most dramatically affected included the "Partnership" clinics in which assigned state employees worked, often at higher salaries, alongside agency employees. All 825 of these state employees were laid off. Eighty percent of the saved salaries were reinvested without fringe benefits in agency contracts. Those who were fortunate enough to transfer to regular employment with the Partnership agencies, typically had to accept pay cuts in the 20% to 40% range (Brotman, 1992). Many others were forced to accept work on a fee-for-service basis under considerably less favorable terms than their former agency or state contracts. Supporters of this move argued that these agencies had been able to "double-dip" because they would bill the state for services performed by the assigned state employees. However, others characterized the layoff as "union busting," pointing out that privatization has typically meant circumventing gains unions had made for state employees.

Two themes pervaded the department's rationale for change in the hospital and community care systems during this period: 1) The system was to be made consumer driven, 2) Public managed care was to be a central organizing principle. These mandates required state administrators to accommodate a Republican governor, generate new revenues, and wrest greater control of the community care system from the unions. The solution consisted of cost shifting, increasing control through privatization using the purchase-of-service system, and adopting the rhetoric of managed competition and managed care. Had the Medicaid program not been simultaneously developing its own mental health system, by using a mainstream managed care strategy, the department may have been able to better adapt managed care to the needs of the mentally ill individuals.

MEDICAID CARVE-OUT PROGRAM: FIRST GENERATION

The focus of this chapter will now shift to the development of the Commonwealth's Medicaid program for the mentally ill—the Massachusetts Mental Health/Substance Abuse Program—during the 1992–96 period, in which the Department of Public Welfare, and later the Division of Medical Assistance, contracted with Mental Health Management of America, Inc., to operate the statewide program under a 1915b HCFA waiver. At the same time that the new program was implemented to provide for the mental health and substance abuse needs of Medicaid recipients, the Department of Mental Health operated a parallel system of services directed at the seriously mentally ill, many of whom were also Medicaid recipients. After an overview of the new Medicaid program, this section will examine its initial implementation, its fine-tuning, and the data available on its impact.

Program Overview

In May 1991 the Massachusetts Department of Public Welfare applied to HCFA for a waiver of selected conditions of Title XIX of the Social Security Act that assure comparability of services and the right of recipients to select their own providers. After a request for additional information, in particular for information to establish that the program would be cost neutral, HCFA granted the waiver for a two-year period beginning in January 1992. The waiver allowed Massachusetts to contract with primary care clinicians to act as gatekeepers and referral sources for each recipient's primary care needs, and to contract with a prepaid health plan to serve as the state's agent for the delivery of mental health and substance abuse services to eligible Medicaid clients (Approval letter, January 30, 1992). Exempt from the program are specialty services such as family planning, AIDS, dental and optical, nursing home, transportation, abortion, and inpatient rehabilitation hospital, and inpatient psychiatric services to persons over age 65 (Massachusetts Department of Public Welfare, 1991, p. 7).

The approval of the 1915b waiver effectively established the MassHealth managed care program. Under this program, all Medicaid recipients must select either one of thirteen health maintenance organizations or a doctor (or nurse practitioner) from the Primary Care Clinician Program. Most of the 5,770 physicians who formerly accepted Medicaid clients were signed up as primary care clinicians. Each of these physicians acts as gatekeeper for all the recipient's medical services, exclusive of exempted services and mental health and substance abuse services. The health maintenance organizations are required to provide the same level of mental health and substance abuse services as the Primary Care Clinician Program, unlike previously when they were required to provide only the standard commercial benefit and the state paid for additional services on a wraparound basis (Bullen, 1995). In contrast, Primary Care Clinician Program recipients receive their mental health services from the Mental Health/Substance Abuse Program as implemented by a private vendor. Because this vendor is a distinct entity vis-à-vis the provider of medical services, the program is regarded as a carved-out program, unlike an integrated program in which the same vendor provides both medical and mental health services.

The Mental Health/Substance Abuse Program was the first such statewide, specialty managed care plan in the nation. Initially, its planners expected to contract with separate providers in each region of the state. After the waiver was first submitted it was decided as part of the request-for-proposals process to select a statewide provider. After review of applications from several major behavioral health companies, state officials selected Mental Health Management of America, Inc. (MHMA), a Tennessee corporation is that is a subsidiary of First Health Services Corporation, which is in turn a subsidiary of First Financial Management Corporation (Fendell, 1994b). Of the state's 656,000 Medicaid recipients, 252,000 were initially enrolled in the Primary Care Clinician and Mental Health/Substance Abuse Programs, whereas 93,000 were enrolled in the health maintenance organizations. The remainder were older adults or person otherwise exempt because they had other forms of insurance (Bullen, 1995, p. 7).

Unlike the fee-for-service Primary Care Clinician Program, the Mental Health/Substance Abuse Program, operated by MHMA, was supported by a type of "soft-capitation" contract in which the state and vendor would share risk (Frank, McGuire, & Newhouse, 1995). Under this plan the vendor would receive an advanced capitated payment for each recipient covered and a somewhat higher payment for each disabled (SSI) recipient. However, the managed care organization paid its providers on a fee-for-service basis. It ended the practice of permitting hospitals to bill separately for room and board, ancillaries, and physician's fees. Comprehensive rates were negotiated instead (Dickey et al., 1995, p. 102). Under this arrangement, HMA was held at risk. However, the contract also contained important incentives. Any unspent revenue was shared with the Division of Medical Assistance/Medicaid, with Medicad retaining 92% and MHMA 8% (Dickey et al., 1995, 102). Under the contract, MHMA could earn $50,000 for each percentage point reduction in hospitalization beyond an agreed upon goal, up to a maximum of $300,000. Later, bonuses for savings to the state were increased to $2 million (Fendell, 1993a, p. 13).

The contract between MHMA and the state was comprehensive. MHMA was required to arrange all acute inpatient treatment, crisis stabilization, outpatient evaluation and treatment, psychiatric day treatment, residential detoxification, and methadone treatment needed by its Medicaid recipients. MHMA was permitted to use diversionary services, such as residential treatment programs, family stabilization, and partial hospitalization. Furthermore, the contract specified that MHMA was also responsible for utilization review, claims processing, systems support, provider relations, and, in general, for decentralized regionally based care management and network management (Dickey et al., 1995, p. 102).

The plan under MHMA was to establish circles of inpatient and outpatient service providers. Recipients were free to see outpatient therapists for up to eight sessions, and after which special approval was needed for extensions. Group therapy was actively promoted, as two ninety-minute sessions were treated as the equivalent of one session of psychotherapy. Responsibility rested on the provider to secure necessary authorization, and unless the provider was turned down outright, the recipient would usually not hear about it (Fendell, 1993b, p. 14). All twenty-four-hour services required prior authorization which was usually valid for only a few days (Callahan, Shepard, Beinecke, Larson, & Cavanaugh, 1995, p. 174). Patients considered extraordinarily violent or who required unusually high levels of service were by policy excluded and referred to a Department of Mental Health facility until their condition improved (Fendell, 1993b, p. 17). Later MHMA contracted with the same crisis intervention/hospital screening teams as the Department of Mental Health did to handle decisions concerning hospital admissions.

Initial Implementation

MHMA commenced its statewide operations in early 1992 through a brief phase-in process. In April it began screening requests for inpatient hospitalizations, and by July it had assumed the role of gatekeeper for outpatient mental health services. Also in July, the partially capitated reimbursement contract between MHMA and the Department of Public Welfare commenced (Fendell, 1993a). At this time the state enrolled 375,000 persons in the MassHealth Program (Callahan et al., 1995, p. 174). A key decision made during this period would later be the basis for an unexpectedly high level of goodwill in the provider community. This was the hiring of almost all staff locally, from among this community. Other tasks accomplished during this period included the development of a provider manual, initial setup of information systems, and establishment of regional offices.

A major problem in implementing the larger MassHealth Program, of which mental health was part, involved securing decisions from each of the recipients as to which health maintenance organization or primary care provider they wished to use. The Department of Public Welfare employed eighty "health benefit managers" to answer questions at an 800 number or by meeting with recipients, as well as providing packets of information. Language barriers were part of the problem. These were ameliorated by assuring that a dozen languages were spoken by the various health benefit managers. Despite the mailings and calls, fewer than half the recipients made an initial choice of provider. Eventually, the department was forced to use a system of computerized assignment, which took into account age, gender, address, language, disability, health, and previous providers. Even so, individual determinations were often required (Bullen, 1995, p. 8). Key issues were how geographic proximity should be weighted vis-à-vis continuity of care, how providers should be paid, what risks providers should have to assume, and who should be responsible for orienting recipients to the new system.

In late 1992 and early 1993, implementation efforts shifted to the formation of a MHMA provider network. According to one Mental Health official, this was perhaps the most politically difficult task in the implementation process. Steps included a formal application process, several surveys, and extensive visits to various facilities. In October, MHMA awarded contracts to forty-five inpatient providers that would be the only facilities eligible for Medicaid reimbursement in other than emergency situations (Dickey et al., 1995, p. 102; Fendell, 1993a). Then, in January 1993, contracts were awarded to outpatient providers. Only a small proportion of applicants were accepted. For example, 465 physicians were selected out of 2,209 applications; 135 clinics out of 263, and 57 hospital outpatient clinics out of 139 (Fendell, 1993a, p. 13). The formation of such provider circles enables the managed care company to purchase services "in bulk" at low rates, and to gain some control over the provider system in exchange for a reduced range of choice on the part of recipients. Also, contracting with a small number of providers, the insurer knows that each provider is more dependent on the insurer's business because a larger percentage of the provider's budget originates from the insurer in a fee-for-service environment.

Another task was the development of the preauthorization and appeals processes. Although these were later improved, providers consistently reported major problems with receiving authorization for services. In addition, there were many problems with the billing and reimbursement systems: MHMA's management information systems appeared to be overwhelmed, payments were often inaccurate, and the prior approval process was a "nightmare" (Beinecke, Goodman, & Rivera, 1995, p. 45). Despite these problems, the number of appeals to MHMA was extremely small, no appeals were filed with the Department of Public Welfare, and no hearings had to be held before the department (Fendell, 1993b, p. 14). Between July and December 1992, there were 528 service denials or diversions. None, however, involved outpatient services. One-half of the informal requests for reconsideration of service denials were reversed. A Department of Public Welfare survey found that two-thirds of the providers expressed some hesitation over appealing MHMA decisions due to concern for their contracts as providers (Fendell, 1992b, p. 14).

Much of the impact of the MHMA program was achieved during the initial year of implementation. During this period, total expenditures were reduced by 22%, supposedly without any reduction in quality or access (Callahan et al., 1995, p. 173). This inflation-adjusted 22% figure is based on a projection of expected increases under the previous fee-for-service program and thus assumes a constant rate of increase. It has been suggested that state officials would have adjusted the rates paid to providers had the new program not been implemented (Fendell, 1993b). Costs declined by about 19% for mental health services, and by 48% for substance abuse services. In both cases, the reduction was attributed to inpatient utilization.

In addition to the decline in inpatient utilization, there was a slight decline in readmission rate, from 19.9% to 18.9%. One study found that the percentage of recipients with one or more hospitalizations decreased from 25.8% in FY 1992 to 14.2% in FY 1993, and those with five or more hospitalizations decreased from 2.0% to 0.4% in the same period (Dickey et al., 1994, p. 109). At the same time, average length of stay in general hospitals dropped from 15.2 to 11.6 days. However, children's readmission rates increased slightly (Callahan et al., 1995, p. 173) at the same time that reports from the field indicated that children were being discharged earlier from hospitals than was the case before the implementation of managed care (Fendell, 1993a). Selected key outpatient services such as outpatient detoxification, clinic treatment, medication, day treatment, clinic evaluation, and methadone counseling were actively promoted (Callahan et. al., 1995, p. 179), although, in aggregate, they diminished slightly during the first year (Dickey et al., 1995, p. 114).

Despite the decline in inpatient utilization, the socioeconomic and diagnostic profile of the recipient population remained essentially unchanged during the first year. Specifically, the disabled did not diminish in number or percentage (Dickey et al., 1995, p. 107). The one unambiguous change was a dramatic increase in substance abuse comorbidity, from 35.6% of recipients to 59.8%. Whether this is a reliable indication of increased substance abuse or of MHMA's encouragement of outpatient substance abuse services remains unclear. Finally, it was also reported that three of four indicators of continuity of care showed improvement (Dickey et al., 1995, p. 107).

Fine-Tuning the Program

Despite initial successes in reducing costs, administrative problems persisted through the remaining three years of the program. These were alleviated somewhat by a redesign of the paperwork, which was applauded by direct service practitioners. In general, outpatient providers liked MHMA's program because it was less rigid and required less paperwork than several other managed care corporations. Some progress in streamlining administrative procedures was attributable to the July 1993 transfer to the state Medicaid program from the Department of Public Welfare to the Division of Medical Assistance. Because the division's overriding responsibility is the administration of Medicare and Medicaid, it was better positioned to manage its contract with MHMA.

During the remaining years of the program, MHMA pursued several initiatives designed to build on the gains made during the first year. In order to minimize problems of coordination with the parallel Department of Mental Health service system, MHMA contracted with the same system of emergency service providers and inpatient crisis units used by Mental Health. In order to enhance the continuity of care, in April 1993 a "primary inpatient psychiatric facility" was designated for each recipient. This policy innovation followed complaints about constant changes of hospital on the part of those recipients who needed frequent hospitalizations.

This same year a "family stabilization team" was initiated to assist families of the seriously mentally ill. Unfortunately, this program never reached more than a token number of recipients and their families. A somewhat better used program was the "intensive case management program," which was established in November 1994 to work with 236 adult and 70 child high users of service. These intensive case managers did not replace Department of Mental Health case managers, even though both systems use a brokerage approach that "tracks and coordinates service delivery and outcomes" (Fendell, 1995a, p. 9). Despite objections from Mental Health concerned about duplication, MHMA proceeded to implement this service (Schaeffler, 1996).

Throughout the implementation and subsequent fine-tuning of the MHMA program, problems of coordination with the state mental health program were sidetracked. Each system had developed its own system of hospitals, case managers, and other providers. Frequently, these systems were duplicative. The two systems, however, used different service categories; for example, MHMA was able to provide a type of partial hospitalization and adolescent residential treatment that the Department of Mental Health was not set up to support (Schaeffler, 1996). The Department of Mental Health's role in coordinating the acute care MHMA system with its own long-term care system was unclear, especially which institution would function as the state mental health authority (Elias & Navon, 1995, p. 49). What limited progress made on these problems was accomplished informally, often between regional and area administrators of the two agencies. It was not until just before termination of the contract with MHMA that these issues were addressed in any systematic manner (see the section "Expansion and Integration of Medicaid Program," below).

Midway through the MHMA contract, the first external evaluation of the program's impact was released in January 1994 by Brandeis University (Callahan, Shepard, Beinecke, Larson, & Cavanaugh, 1994). Because the Department of Public Welfare had contracted for both this and a second evaluation (Beneicke, Goodman, & Rivera, 1995) within an extremely limited budget, it was impossible for either research team to conduct either a client satisfaction or outcome component. They relied on an analysis of existing databases, as well as on a survey of administrators of provider agencies. As a result, the project produced a favorable report but one that amplified a few of MHMA's administrative problems. The report received only lukewarm reviews from the advocacy community. Its failure to survey consumers exemplified to many the general lack of consumer involvement in the program (Fendell, 1994a). Some pointed out that the positive report from providers may actually represent a measurement problem: "Off the record, medical professionals at hospitals and clinics report fear of retaliation for direct or indirect criticism of MHMA" (Fendell, 1994a). The Division of Medical Assistance conducted its own survey of 2,000 consumers, which reportedly revealed a high level of satisfaction ("Massachusetts Announces," 1995). One of the few changes to come out of the Brandeis evaluation was a push on the part of the division to have MHMA develop a quality assurance program, which it subsequently did (Schaeffler, 1996).

Overall Impact of Program

Two external evaluations of the MHMA program have been conducted, and neither was able to assess its impact on recipients (Beinecke et al., 1995; Callahan et al., 1995); although the internal Division of Medical Assistance survey did find an overall level of consumer satisfaction ("Massachusetts Announces," 1995). However, there is considerably more information available from these evaluations on the program's impact on service delivery patterns and costs.

During the first year, the MHMA program lead to a 2.4% reduction in hospitalization levels from the previous year, from 16.5 users per 1,000 enrollees to 16.1 (see table 1). This level remained fairly constant in the following years, at 16.2 for 1994, and reportedly at similar levels in FY 1995 and

TABLE 1   Utilization Levels for Mental Health and Substance Abuse Services under the MHMA Program, 1992–1994 (users per 1,000 enrollees)

Service Type	1992	1993	1994
Mental health			
Inpatient mental health	16.5	16.1	16.2
Clinic treatment	118.5	131.2	141.7
Clinic evaluation	67.5	70.8	77.1
Outpatient (hospital)	59.7	48.7	44.5
Psychiatrists	32.5	28.6	27.4
Clinic medication	24.7	31.9	42.3
Crisis intervention	18.3	15.9	17.3
Psychologists	16.3	11.5	11.7
Home care	6.0	5.4	n.a.
Psychiatric day treatment	3.7	4.7	3.9
Clinic consultation	0.00	38.3	41.9
Acute residential (children)	0.01	1.3	1.8
Community health center	6.0	5.4	5.9
Substance abuse			
Inpatient	9.1	3.5	0.9
Freestanding detoxification	5.5	7.9	9.2
Level III detoxification	0.0	2.4	3.4
Acute residential	0.0	3.2	4.7
Outpatient	9.6	9.2	9.7
Methadone counseling	5.4	6.2	7.5
Methadone dosing	5.2	6.3	7.6
Acute residential (children/adolescents)	0.0	0.1	0.2
Total, all services	212.7	222.6	n.a.

SOURCES: 1992 and 1993—J. J. Callahan, Jr., et al., "Evaluation of the Massachusetts Medicaid Mental Health/Substance Abuse Program," Heller School for Advanced Studies in Social Welfare, Brandeis University, January 24, 1994; 1994—R. Beinecke et al., "An Assessment of the Massachusetts Managed Mental Health/Substance Abuse Program: Year Three," Department of Public Management, Suffolk University, May 1995.

FY 1996 (Fendell, 1996). Some observers complained about a scarcity of diversionary beds, though there were more beds than before ("Massachusetts Achieves," 1995). In substance abuse there were particularly dramatic shifts, as inpatient care dropped from 9.1 users per 1,000 enrollees to 3.5 in the first year, and then to 0.9 by the second year (Beinecke et al., 1995; Callahan et al., 1995).

More dramatic shifts in services took place in community programs, specifically those dispensing medications. Although MHMA and Division of Medical Assistance had promised to increase outpatient care in light of their plan to reduce inpatient services, utilization of outpatient services actually declined from 59.7 users per 1,000 enrollees to 48.7 in the first year and 44.5 in the second year. One report claimed a 6% increase in the number of enrollees receiving only outpatient treatment. However, this no doubt reflects the even greater reductions in hospital and other services ("Massachusetts Achieves," 1995). By 1994, the decline in outpatient utilization was reported to have stabilized (Fendell, 1994b). In contrast, an initial population of 4,000 persons in July 1992 who took psychiatric medications ballooned to 7,500 by September 1995 (Fendell, 1995b), an 87.5% increase. Similarly, the Brandeis report found a 29.1% increase in medication utilization during the first year, from 24.7 to 31.9, while the Beinecke study found a subsequent 32.6% increase in the second year, from 31.9 to 42.3 (Beinecke et al., 1995; Callahan et al., 1995).

The increase in psychiatric medications was paralleled by dramatic increases in methadone dosing and counseling in the substance abuse arena. Methadone dosing increased from 5.2 users per 1,000 enrollees to 6.3 in the first year and 7.6 in the second, or 46.2% in the first two years of the program; methadone counseling increased almost as much over the same period, from 5.4 to 7.5, or 38.9%. Similarly, freestanding detoxification also grew dramatically, from 5.5 to 9.2 in these two years, or 67.3%. Psychotherapeutically oriented practitioners may have historically been especially cautious regarding the use of psychiatric or other mind-altering drugs. However, cost-conscious MHMA managers no doubt saw major gains to be made through the promotion of these therapies. Whether the optimum level of medication usage is closer to the baseline or the later levels is a question that only a consumer outcome study can answer.

A key component to community care is crisis intervention. Levels clearly decreased, from 18.3 users per 1,000 enrollees to 15.9, or 13.5%, in the first year then went back up to 17.3 in the second year, a 8.8% correction (Beinecke et al., 1995; Callahan et al., 1995). One report indicated that the growth in the second year continued at a "dramatic" pace in the program's third year (Fendell, 1995b).

After initial growth of day program utilization in the first year, from 3.7 users per 1,000 enrollees to 4.7, a rise of 27%, utilization in the second year returned almost to its original level, 3.9. According to more recent data, utilization levels fell 20% between July 1992 and October 1994 (Fendell, 1995a).

Officials have pointed out dramatic increases in other areas of community programming, but by 1996 each of these areas could claim only minimal enrollment of Medicaid recipients. When actual enrollment levels are examined, these changes consisted of increases from very to extremely low levels of utilization. For instance, out of 373,000 enrollees in spring 1996, only 19 were receiving community support, 1 flex benefits, 17 partial hospitalization, and 203 crisis stabilization (Fendell, 1996). With the exception of medication, virtually every area of community care saw a decrease in service utilization. Because of the dramatic increase in the prescription of psychiatric medication during the first year of the program, overall levels of service utilization remained fairly constant, increasing only slightly, from 212.7 to 222.6, or 4.6%. Unfortunately, no data are reported on the average length of stay or number of units of service used, except for inpatient care, where average length of stay leveled off. None of the evaluations attempted to assess the reliability of the data or the statistical significance of the shifts in service utilization.

Limited data are available on the impact of the foregoing service patterns on subpopulations such as children and the disabled. MHMA did significantly decrease length of stay in twenty-four-hour facilities: for children and adolescents by 29.8% between FY 1992 and FY 1993 and for adults by 10.3%. At the time, the readmission rate was increasing among children. Shepard, one of the Brandeis investigators, suggested that this was mainly the result of the Massachusetts child welfare agency's practice of "parking kids in hospitals" ("Massachusetts Achieves," 1995). However, the Brandeis study reported that for the first year the nondisabled were more seriously affected than the disabled.

Fendell, who reviewed data on the remaining years of the program, concluded that disabled recipients experienced larger cuts in mental health clinic and hospital outpatient therapy. Between June 1992 and May 1995, the number of disabled recipients seen by clinics declined by 133%, and those seen by hospital clinics by 15%. Similarly, units of treatment rendered to disabled recipients by hospital clinics dropped by 25% (Fendell, 1995b, p. 13). This decline occurred at the same time that 79% of providers noted in one survey that their clients were more severely disturbed than the year before (FY 1993; Beinecke et al., 1995, p. 29). Overall, the preponderance of evidence suggests that the disabled—those on SSI—were disproportionately affected by reductions in services.

Some of the evaluations examined the program's impact on the quality of administrative decision making. In one study, one-tenth of the providers (10%) rated the review process excellent, while slightly over half (53%) rated it very good, 28% good, 6% fair, and 3% poor (Beinecke et al., 1995, p. 37). In general, MHMA was considered to be about the same or slightly better than other managed care corporations with respect to quality of utilization review decisions, access for clients, flexibility, and promptness in making decisions (Callahan et al., 1995, p. 181). One provider noted that

The Medicaid carve-out has been fairly cooperative and collegial versus adversarial and oppositional. My feeling is that the people who have been hired to do this were reasonably knowledgeable regarding the state and sensitive in terms of access to treatment by a more disabled population and not restricting the provider network. ("Massachusetts Achieves," 1995)

The managed care program has also had some impact on service organizations and administration at the provider level, although much of this impact is no doubt a response to the general infusion of managed care increased competition into the service community. In the Beiecke study almost half the providers reported that they had recently merged with, acquired, or otherwise affiliated with one or more other organizations (1995, p. 181). These actions are intended to reduce overhead costs and enhance the provider's attractiveness to managed care companies. Virtually all of the providers (94%) said they had increased measurement of services and outcomes; over two-thirds (71%) expanded or improved their management information systems; and most (84%) added or strengthened internal gatekeeper and utilization review functions (p. 51). Some of these developments have been specifically linked with the state's use of detailed contracting specifications and reporting requirements on access, service expenditures, and consumer compliance ("Massachusetts Achieves," 1995).

Since a key rationale for the Medicaid managed care program was that it would save money, or at least be cost neutral, each of the evaluations examined costs. Both concluded that substantial savings were achieved, but mostly during the start-up period (Beinecke et al., 1995, p. 25; Callahan et al., 1995). The greatest savings were achieved by diverting hospital admissions from inpatient services to outpatient care, particularly in substance abuse, and by negotiating substantial price reductions with hospitals (Frank et al., 1995, p. 53). It is reported that between June 1992 and May 1995 per recipient expenditures fell by 44%, for children by 53% (Fendell, 1995b, p., 14). Nonetheless, outpatient expenditures also declined, in part because reimbursement rates did not rise as fast as inflation ("Massachusetts Achieves," 1995, p. 4). However, in specific areas there were substantial cost increases, as would be expected from the earlier review of service trends. These include crisis care and medication prescription (Fendell, 1995a, 1996). It should be pointed out that both the Brandeis and Beinecke evaluations were premised on the assumption that had the previous program continued, costs would have continued to rise in a straight-line fashion, and, this predicted level was used as the baseline from which cost savings of the new program were calculated.

Overall, the formal evaluations found that the program saved money and maintained access and quality of services. These studies only focused on the first two years of the program, and many of the trends identified did not hold up in the third and fourth years. The only consistent increase in community services throughout the period appears to have been in medication utilization. While initially there were increases in crisis care, even this subsided by the end of the program. Unfortunately, neither of these studies provided data that were directly relevant to quality of services. Both relied on service providers rating their own quality in a time of diminishing resources and competitiveness for managed care contracts, hardly a convincing or reassuring methodology. In addition, no data have been collected on any consumer outcomes other than recidivism rates. Thus, while some data suggest cost savings, the data on service trends suggest reduced utilization of most types of services, except medication prescription. Despite overall provider approval of MHMA, one of the most frequent complaints of the advocacy community has been its failure to share information. This criticism perhaps illustrates one of the central limitations of privatized oversight of services, that policy decisions and resulting trends become increasingly inaccessible, thereby crippling the ability of advocates to monitor the system.

EXPANSION AND INTEGRATION OF MEDICAID PROGRAM

During 1995 and 1996, the Medicaid program was expanded on two fronts. The first involved recontracting with the Mental Health/Substance Abuse Program, managed by MHMA, until June 30, 1996. In its recontracting, the program was expanded to include acute care services previously contracted by the Department of Mental Health. The second involved an 1115 HCFA waiver that consolidated several programs and in general expanded Medicaid coverage to almost all low-income persons without medical insurance.

Expansion in the Mental Health/Substance Abuse Carve-Out Program

Through the four years of the MHMA program, the Department of Mental Health and Department of Public Welfare/Division of Medical Assistance had no formal written agreement about their respective areas of oversight responsibility. In September 1995, the Department of Mental Health and the Division of Medical Assistance signed a statement of understanding that committed these agencies to developing an interagency agreement resolving the various problems inherent in the state's operating two public mental health systems.

After several drafts and numerous public hearings, the interagency agreement was signed in spring 1996. The agreement preserved the notion of two separate systems but attempted to reduce areas of overlap by defining the Department of Mental Health continuing care and the Division of Medical Assistance/Medicaid system as one involving acute care. This distinction was defined by the transfer of Mental Health funds to Medical Assistance for contracted services for short-term inpatient crisis units with private general hospitals and for crisis intervention and other diversionary services with agencies. In turn, the Division of Medical Assistance agreed to use these funds to contract with the managed care organization (MHMA) for these same services. In exchange, about 30,000 Mental Health–eligible consumers, whether Medicaid recipients or not, would receive acute care services through the Division of Medical Assistance's managed care system. Long-term and intermediate care hospital and community-based services would continue to be directly managed by the Department of Mental Health ("Massachusetts Announces," 1995). The interagency agreement also formalized a role for the department in establishing and monitoring the contract with the managed care organization as well as a role for the Division of Medical Assistance in overseeing certain Department of Mental Health responsibilites.

Many in the advocacy community, as well as many providers and some state officials, have questioned the logic of dichotomizing the system into acute and continuing care and the practicality of implementing the labyrinthine agreement intended to coordinate them. To many, it provides too many opportunities for state officials to "pass the buck" and, in general, prescribes too many convoluted administrative procedures to be effective. However, the mental health commissioner at that time, Eileen Elias, argued that "this agreement will end the two-tier system of mental health service delivery that has existed for too long. More importantly, it will fulfill the vision and promise of the community mental health movement" ("Massachusetts Announces," 1995).

Massachusetts was the first state to pursue a joint purchasing agreement on such a scale between its state mental health authority and Medicaid agency ("Massachusetts Announces," 1995). The initial idea for this second-generation program was reported to have originated from Commissioner Elias after she learned of Medicaid takeovers of state mental health authority services in other states. Concerned about this possibility, she initiated discussions with the medical assistance commissioner about a formal agreement in which the Department of Mental Health would turn over designated services but retain some control. The central means for the implementation of the agreement involved a request for proposals for the renewal of the contract between the Division of Medical Assistance and its managed care organization, until this time, MHMA, dated September 22, 1995. Most observers had assumed that MHMA would have its contract renewed. Despite vocal consumer concerns about MHMA, an interagency review committee was reported to have supported contract renewal for MHMA. However, the state did not accept this recommendation. Instead, it negotiated a contract for the third-ranked alternative, a joint application by Options Mental Health and Value Mental Health. Together, they formed the Massachusetts Behavioral Health Partnership (MBHP, or "the Partnership"). Unsuccessful appeals from other applicants slowed the signing of the new contract until only two days prior to its start date of July 1, 1996. The reasons the state did not select MHMA have not been divulged. One further development, however, may indicate a possible reason. In the final months of the MHMA contract, there were reportedly major cost overruns, which resulted in a lawsuit filed by Mental Health Corporations of Massachusetts on behalf of MHMA providers. This lawsuit resulted in a settlement in which MHMA agree to pay its vendors 70% of outstanding balances (Schaeffler, 1996).

An even more complicated system of incentives and disincentives have reportably been built into the contract with the new managed care organization. It attempts to put more of the responsibility for the costs of mental health services on federal and other non-state-funded programs (Fendell, 1995b, p. 13). It also relaxes human rights requirements in contracts for short-term hospital units and allows hospitals to develop their own human rights protocols "consistent" with Department of Mental Health human rights policy (Fendel, 1995b, p. 12). In addition, it includes sanctions designed to improve discharge planning and to reduce untimely inpatient admissions, inappropriate referrals to Mental Health continuing care services, delayed prior approvals and payments to providers, and late submission of reports to the state (Fendell, 1995b). Unlike in the former contract, the new contract specifically allows the use of capitation funding from the managed care organization to its providers in the third year of the contract. MBHP's new provider manual suggests these cost pressures were being passed through this system to clients. For instance, among the criteria for eligible clients are the stipulations that "individuals must demonstrate response/improvement to treatment as a condition to its continuation" and "individuals must demonstrate compliance (medication and program) or they shall not receive services" (Flory, 1996, pp. 5–6). In light of the incentive structures developed, Brotman's comment—that "the criteria for choosing a successor is being driven increasingly by downward pricing pressure, which could have a negative impact on the chronically disabled"—is particularly insightful ("Massachusetts Achievers," 1995).

Overall Expansion: The 1115 Waiver Program

From 1994 to 1995, Commissioner Bruce Bullen of the Division of Medical Assistance had a team developing an application for a second, extended federal waiver program. Laurie Burgess, the director of this group, reported that the largest barrier was the need to demonstrate that extensions of the program would ultimately be budget neutral ("Health Care Reform," 1994). The final waiver application developed and submitted called for the extension of Medicaid to 75% of the currently uninsured persons with incomes below 200% of the federal poverty level and to virtually everyone with incomes below 133% of the poverty level ("Health Care Reform," 1994). This would include most Department of Mental Health non-Medicaid consumers as well as virtually all the homeless. In addition, it calls for several health care programs, such as the Medical Security Plan for the short-term unemployed and

CommonHealth Plan for the disabled, to be folded into the MassHealth program. It consisted of the option of either a health maintenance organization or the Primary Care Clinician and Mental Health/Substance Abuse Programs. There would be a single conclusion form for all state medical assistance programs. Besides the program consolidations, other funding would arise from savings gained through the increased use of managed care and of small state assistance programs ("Massachusetts Medicaid," 1995).

The federal government approved the 1115 waiver application on April 24, 1995 ("MassHealth Waiver," 1995). Almost immediately (April 28, 1996) Governor Weld filed the state legislation required to make the waiver program part of a more comprehensive health care reform package, which was sent to the Special Commission of Health Care. Approved by this group in September 1995, the legislation was forwarded to the Massachusetts House Ways and Means Committee. After being consolidated with other health reform legislation, the reform package was passed by the legislature and signed by the governor in July 1996. The act was contingent on further study to assure that the program in total would be cost neutral. This study was completed in fall 1996 and demonstrated either cost neutrality or savings for all but one implementation scenario. As a result, it was planned that the implementation of the waiver would begin by July 1997. Although Governor Weld supported the program, he subsequently backed off supporting the component that would insure all children in families with incomes between 133% and 200% of the poverty level ("Weld Balks," 1996). Despite uncertainty about the implementation of the children's component, it has survived as the only part to be implemented as of February 1998.

CONCLUSION

At its inception, managed care embodied a range of ideals involving the integration of service delivery. However, due to pressures for cost containment, managed care in mental health has come to be regarded primarily as a tool of cost saving. A primary means for such saving has been cost shifting, the transfer of service costs to other sources, most recently to the federal government through the Medicaid waiver process and the further privatization of service delivery, and especially of service oversight.

In Massachusetts, the management of mental health care has a long history. Only since the early 1990s, however, has the rhetoric of managed care in Department of Mental Health efforts been supplanted with its actuality under Medicaid leadership. Because of this rhetoric, as well as Mental Health's most recent privatization efforts, the stage was set for Medicaid to assume control of important mental health services in the current second-generation carveout program. Beyond the transfer of control of acute Department of Mental Health services, the most important change has been the extended privatization of the department's oversight functions under Medicaid auspices. In the first-generation program these changes meant a medicalization of mental health services and a retreat from a comprehensive continuum of care, including psychiatric rehabilitative programs, to increasing reliance on medication. It also meant the fragmentation of professional decision making. While costs were reduced, partly through cost shifting, achievement of managed care's ideal of service integration has been sidetracked by political and economic accommodations.

This author has yet to hear a serious argument from any of the constituents of the current dichotomized system of acute and continuing managed health care in Massachusetts that such a split will improve the integration of service delivery. Given that managed care is being implemented, the critical question is whether a separate, carved-out system for disabled populations, such as the long-term mentally ill, will better protect their interests than an attempt to merge them into mainstream managed care organizations, such as health maintenance organizations. This question has only served to distract from the equally important question of the role of the state mental health authority in managing the service system. However, both problems become particularly urgent now that most of the long-term mentally ill, who formerly did not have Medicaid coverage, are enrolled in the Medicaid system under the 1115 waiver program in Massachusetts, and no doubt soon will be in other states.

REFERENCES

Beinecke, R. H., Goodman, M., & Rivera, M. (1995, May). *An assessment of the Massachusetts managed Mental Health/Substance Abuse Program: Year three.* Boston: Suffolk University, Department of Public Management.

Brotman, A. (1992). Privatization of mental health services: The Massachusetts experiment. *Journal of Health Politics, Policy and Law,* 17(3), 541–551.

Bullen, B. M. (1995, Spring). Managed care in Massachusetts. *Public Welfare,* 53(4), 6–9.

Callahan, J. J. Shepard, D. S., Beinecke, R. H., Larson, M. J., & Cavanaugh, D. (1994, January). Evaluation of the Massachusetts Medicaid Mental Health/Substance Abuse Program. Unpublished manuscript, Brandeis University, Heller School for Advanced Studies in Social Welfare.

Callahan, J. J., Shepard, D. S., Beinecke, R. H., Larson, M. J., & Cavanaugh, D. (1995). Mental health/substance abuse treatment in managed care: The Massachusetts Medicaid experience. *Health Affairs,* 14(3), 173–84.

Dickey, B., Norton, E. C., Normand, S.-L., Axeni, H., Fisher, W., & Altaffer, F. (1995). Massachusetts Medicaid managed health care reform: Treatment for the psychiatrically disabled. In J. C. Cantor, R. M. Scheffler, and L. F. Rossiter (Eds.), *Advances in health economics and health services research.* Greenwich, CT: JAI.

Dowart, R. A., & Epstein, S. S. (1993). *Privatization and mental health care: A fragile balance.* Westport, CT: Auburn.

Elias, E., & Navon, M. (1995). The Massachusetts experience with managed mental health care and Medicaid. *Health Affairs, 14*(3), 46–49.

Essock, S. M., & Goldman, H. H. (1995). States' embrace of managed mental health care. *Health Affairs, 14*(3), 34–44.

Fendell, S. (1993a, March). Managed care in the Medicaid mental health system: Verdict out, concerns abound. *Advisor* (Mental Health Legal Advisors Committee), pp. 10–15.

Fendell, S. (1993b, Fall). Mental health managed care: Service expenditures down MHMA profits up. *Advisor,* pp. 14–17, 30–35.

Fendell, S. (1994a, Spring). Mental health managed care: MHMA report card mixed; conflict between profits and consumers. *Advisor,* pp. 4–12.

Fendell, S. (1994b, Fall). Managed care update. *Advisor,* pp. 9–16.

Fendell, S. (1995a, Spring). Managed care initiative expands; impact continues to be felt. *Advisor,* pp. 8–16.

Fendell, S. (1995b, Fall). Mental health managed care: Expansion to DMH acute care and Medicaid update. *Advisor,* pp. 12–15.

Fendell, S. (1996, Spring). Managed care trends. *Advisor,* p. 9.

Flory, B. (1996, July/August). How will Massachusetts' managed care initiative meet the needs of individuals with severe mental illness? Marblehead, MA: Alliance for the Mentally Ill of the North Shore.

Frank, R. G., McGuire, T. G., & Newhouse, J. P. (1995). Risk contracts in managed mental health care. *Health Affairs, 14*(3), 50–64.

Health care reform waiver nears decision. (1994). *The DMA newsletter, 1*(2).

Hudson, C. G., Flory, C. B., III, & Friedrich, R. M. (1995, February 1). Trends in psychiatric hospitalization and long term care: A plan for ongoing monitoring and advocacy. Marblehead, MA: National Alliance for the Mentally Ill, Hospital and Long Term Care Network.

Hudson, C. G., Salloway, J. C., & Vissing, Y. M. (1992). The impact of state administrative practices on community mental health. *Administration and Policy in Mental Health, 19*(6), 417–436.

Iglehart, J. K. (1996). Managed care and mental health. *New England Journal of Medicine, 334*(2), 131–135.

Leadholm, B. A., & Kerzner, J. P. (1995). Public managed care: Comprehensive community support in Massachusetts. *Administration and Policy in Mental Health, 22*(5), 543–552.

Manderscheid, R. W., and Sonnenschein, M. A. (Eds.). (1990). *Mental health: United States, 1990.* Center of Mental Health Services and National Institute of Mental Health, (DHHS Publication No. SMA 90–1708). Washington, DC: Government Printing Office.

Massachusetts achieves success in moving to managed Medicaid. (1995). *Psychiatric News, 80*(24), 7.

Massachusetts announces Medicaid/mental health partnership. (1994, Fall). *DMA Newsletter, 2*(2), 4.

Massachusetts Department of Mental Health. (1985, December). Comprehensive plan to improve services for chronically mentally ill persons. Boston: Author.

Massachusetts Department of Mental Health (1993, January). Developing a system of public managed care: A progress report. Boston: Author.

Massachusetts Department of Public Welfare. (1991, May). Massachusetts Medicaid managed care program (MassCare)—Section 1915(B) waiver request. Boston: Author.

Massachusetts Medicaid waiver portends broader coverage. (1995). *Hospital and Health Networks, 69*(11), 12.

MassHealth waiver program goes to special commission. (1995). *DMA Newsletter, 2*(1), 9.

Schaeffler, C. Deputy Commissioner for Program Operations, Massachusetts Department of Mental Health. (1996, August 2). Interview.

"Weld balks at Medicaid expansion." (1995, January 12). *Boston Globe*, p. A20.

Wisor, R. L., Jr. (1993). Community care, competition and coercion: A legal perspective on privatized mental health care. *American Journal of Law and Medicine, 19*(1, 2), 145–176.

CHAPTER 5

Redesigning a Community-Based System of Child and Family Services

Barbara Thomlison
Professor, School of Social Work, Florida International University

William Meade
Chief Executive Officer, Calgary Rockyview Child and Family Authority

James Pritchard
Director of Community Services, Hull Community Services, Calgary

The Alberta government is launching a community-based system of child and family services. This will involve the formation of seventeen child and family services authorities to oversee the planning and delivery of services to children and families in Alberta communities. As a current program implementation in process, not all elements of the emerging model are in place or negotiated. This case study examines the process and structure of redesigning a public system of children's services into a community-governed, nonprofit, voluntary, private sector managed system of local service networks.

The context leading to the service system planning, its design process, and a description of the emerging model for the service system is identified. Stakeholder participation and local community governance were the hallmarks of the new service system. Quality is emphasized in the process and structure of the new system and is seen as the involvement of all stakeholders from the community in all aspects of the planning, design, delivery, and impact of services. The people and structures critical to the redesigned service system are described.

CANADIAN CONTEXT OF CHILDREN'S SERVICES

Canada, an officially bilingual nation, has a population of 30 million people living under a unique system of governmentally "subsidized capitalism" that is a foundation for a liberal social welfare system. Child welfare services in Canada are a provincially mandated responsibility with each province having its own child and family services legislation and service delivery model. Legislation, financing, government monitoring, voluntary collaboration, and social worker education, training, and experience also vary across provinces. Some provinces, such as Ontario, mandate children's services through a system of children's aid societies, while others, such as British Columbia and Alberta, provide the same program through centrally controlled government-delivered services. Each province tends to honor the major principles of least intrusive interventions, family support for protection and safety of children, permanency planning, and, wherever possible, nonadversarial approaches through family preservation ideology. Services are expected to contribute supports and resources promoting family autonomy and independence.

Families needing assistance from multiple service systems are recognized as requiring long-term help in caring for their children (Ministry of Supply and Services, 1994). There are approximately 50,000 children in permanent out-of-home care in Canada. Minority groups, such as aboriginal, blacks, and Asians, are overrepresented in the out-of-home care population compared to their distribution in the population. Some communities have developed special agencies to provide services to these populations.

The Case for a New Focus in Alberta

Although Alberta consists of large rural sectors and an economy based on ranching and exploration of natural resources, its population of approximately three million is concentrated in a few cities. The province has a tradition of political conservatism, an entrepreneurial approach to the spectrum of fiscal and social issues, and a private-public mix of efforts. Alberta's annual governmental spending on children and youth, including health, education, justice, and family and social services totals $2,326,55 million (Canada West Foundation, 1996). Family and social services receive approximately 13% of these funds. A powerful, politically conservative public supports fiscal viability of social, health, and educational services by remolding the social welfare system and reducing government expenditures.

Child and Family Services Context.   Historically, the government of Alberta has provided child and family services within six geographic areas through a mixed model of regional autonomy and centralized policy making, including budgeting, policy formulation, and standard setting for service delivery. Centralized authority and responsibility were thought to provide throughout the province for service delivery, resource allocation and practice standards (Rothery, Gallup, Tillman, & Allard, 1995; Thomlison, 1984). However, this model of governance has been repeatedly criticized for political- and managerial-based decisions that did not take into account local and community-based needs (Mackenzie, 1991; Thomlison, 1984). These criticisms include lack of sensitivity and indifference to regional issues and diversity dilemmas as well as inequitable distribution of resources.

Child Protection.   Protection services were needed for 7,109 children, with approximately 4,000 Alberta children in out-of-home care (Ministry of Supply and Services, 1994). The province has a rising population of older youth in care (30% are age 15 or older) who have complex, multifaceted problems that require long-term services from numerous systems such as special education, mental health, juvenile justice, vocational education, and child welfare. Direct care services, such as placement, treatment, and support programs were regionally planned and managed through service contracts to a combination of the nonprofit and private sectors of the community. Concerns for the out-of-home care population include issues of continuity and quality of care.

Although the aboriginal child population makes up only 1% of the general child population in Alberta, it represents 50% of the out-of-home care population. Currently, there are several agreements enabling the aboriginal communities to deliver their own child welfare services. Where there are no formal agreements, provincial government staff are responsible for delivering child protection services.

A two-year review of public child and family services structures by the provincial Children's Advocate grew out of child fatalities and other serious negative outcomes for children receiving services (Alberta Children's Advocate, 1993). This review was conducted against the background of public pressure to reduce costs and improve standards of care and enhance practice effectiveness. The final report recommended the redesign of services. The change initiative was mandated in 1994. The goal was to devise a structure to oversee and efficiently delivery a broad array of services to children and families in Alberta, thereby changing the role and relationship between government and the community.

Planning for the Process

The change initiative was launched when the government of Alberta issued a report, "Focus on Children" (Alberta Family and Social Services, 1994), which announced the mandate to improve child and family services. The shift from a government-delivered services system to one built on stakeholder participation and local community governance was to occur within three years. Integrated services, community-based services, improved aboriginal services, and a focus on early intervention were four pillars for planning the service networks.

The process for the change would emerge through the newly created Office of the Provincial Commissioner of Services for Children (Alberta Family and Social Services, 1994). Local Offices of the Commissioner of Services for Children and Families were established throughout the province to coordinate the community initiative in each of seventeen newly designated regions.

In November 1994, the Interdepartmental Deputy and Assistant Deputy Ministers Committee was formed by the minister of family and social services. Representing the ministries of Family and Social Services, Health, Justice, Education, Community Development, and Aboriginal Affairs and the Alberta Alcohol and Drug Abuse Commission, this group was to provide leadership to the community-based initiatives and specifically address policy issues that span and influence these intertwined child-serving systems as the process unfolded.

CALGARY ROCKYVIEW EXPERIENCE

Table 1 summarizes the key accomplishment in the process of the Calgary Rockyview Children's Services Redesign Initiative, one of the seventeen regional community initiatives. The rest of this chapter examines in detail the Rockyview experience.

The Community: Calgary Rockyview Region

In 1994 Calgary initiated an inclusive community planning process through the local Office of the Commissioner of Services for Children and Families focusing on the desired structures, mechanisms, and outcomes for children, families, and community. A regional director of planning and development and a total of seven community facilitators, two of whom were aboriginal, staffed the office. The community facilitators worked directly with groups, neighborhoods, and communities to document their input, ideas, and planning suggestions.

An inclusive community planning process was the vision. The planning process was to:

include a wide range as well as a cross section of stakeholders to identify and solve issues,

follow a consensus decision-making style,

use group meetings in the consensus decision-making strategies, and

encourage citizens and members of power structures to collaborate on the redesign planning process.

While the redesign plan outlined many generic features, participants and stakeholders were expected to adapt or create a planning approach that identified and responded to the needs of their localities.

TABLE 1 Timeline of Calgary Rockyview Children's Service Redesign Initiative
1993–94

1993–1994	Commissioner appointed
	Provincial community consultation
1994	Report: "Focus on Children"
	Announcement of redesign initiative
1995	Zone 4 community presentations
	24 Working groups formed
	Acting steering committee formed
	Vision Circle developed
1996	Preliminary service plan developed from working group
	Submissions
	Focus groups, surveys
	5 Service domains identified
	Design groups formed
1997	Service integration teams put together the domain planning
	Steering committee takes service plan to commissioner
1998	Child and family services authority established
	Regional authority develops business plan
May 1998	Regional child and family services authority in operation

Situation Assessment

Involving system stakeholders as participants in the planning process began with a situation assessment, which analyzed community needs in detail, and identified the resources and supports needed to address these needs. Community forums and meetings were organized to stimulate community and stakeholder interest and participant support for the initial situation assessment review. This part of the process had four elements: 1) zone community presentation, 2) formation of twenty-four community working groups, 3) creation of a Children and Family Services Steering Committee, and 4) development of the mission statement—the Vision Circle.

1. Zone Community Presentation, February–April 1995. A series of public presentations were conducted across the Calgary Rockyview Region by the staff of the Office of the Commissioner of Services for Children and Families. The presentations were to address two questions: Why there is a need to change the system? Who is to do the planning? These presentations were also seen as opportunity to invite the widest possible range of stakeholder groups to participate in the planning process.

2. Twenty-Four Community Working Groups, April 1995. Twenty-four working groups were formed following the zone community presentations and included everyone who expressed an interest in participating in the situation assessment. Working groups were charged with determining vision, goals, outcomes, and action plans for an array of services for children and families. The working groups formed around major interest themes, including family violence, children with special needs, aboriginal services, day care services, children in long-term care, aggressive children, crisis services, and geographic localities. Membership in the community working groups was diverse in terms of interests, concerns, and expression of need for involvement. The twenty-four working groups were composed of several hundred participants from various sectors who met one or two times per month throughout the first year of the planning process.

Community working groups began with the task of assessing the situation and needs of children, families, and communities using a self-assessment community workbook (Alberta Commission of Services, 1995). Part of the assessment entailed a review of what stakeholders thought was working effectively and what elements of service organization and delivery they thought needed improvement.

The assessment also addressed the extent to which the existing strategies and services were congruent with the emerging service plan. This component sought ways the existing services could be reshaped to support the intent of the community consensus-building process. For example, working groups proposed strategies and ways of determining the level of intervention needed to divert families from adversarial service approaches. To allow for a wider mix of services emphasizing early intervention and family support perspectives, it was determined that a decrease in crisis and protection services was needed.

3. Calgary Rockyview Children and Family Services Steering Committee, May 1995.   The aims of this interim organization were to oversee the planning process and to advise on the direction and conditions for both the planning process and new structure as they emerged. Both in membership and purpose it was charged to have the widest community-based support and participation possible. It served as the predecessor to the permanent structure, the regional child and family services authority. The media was used to solicit volunteers and nominations for cochairs (one aboriginal cochair was deemed important) as well as for members of the steering committee. The provincial minister of family and social services appointed the steering committee from applications submitted.

This eighteen-member steering committee completed a two-year term and provided a linkage between the provincial government and the Calgary Rockyview community. Committee membership included the director of the City Social Services Department, a deputy chief superintendent from a school board, the dean of the Faculty of Social Work from the University of Calgary, a member of the regional health authority, six aboriginal members representing services and consumers of service, a director of a local parent support organization, and a young adult who is the former director of a youth-in-care organization. There was one rural citizen representative from the region of Rockyview. Both the cochairs were from the private sector of the community and came with extensive experience in the voluntary sector.

Over the next two years, the steering committee met extensively and organized numerous large town meetings of the community. Members viewed themselves as "keepers of the process" and not as a group of experts. The Children and Family Services Steering Committee related directly to the working groups and the community as a whole. The steering committee was supported by the local Office of the Commissioner of Services for Children and Families through the community facilitators.

4. Mission Statement: The Vision Circle, June 1995. Based on a town hall gathering of the community, the Children and Family Services Steering Committee integrated the various statements, submissions, and desired directions of the twenty-four working groups into one document called the Vision Circle (see figure 1). The Vision Circle has become a strong, identifiable symbol among the stakeholders and represents the values and principles for the new service system and its implementation. The Vision Circle places the child at the center, surrounded by specific outcomes and supports. Outcomes include safety, self-worth, capable, loved, and belonging. To sustain children in their families and communities, supports must be provided that are flexible, sustainable, personalized, accountable, compassionate, and responsive. The community, consisting of funders, cultural groups, businesses, and friends, provides supports. To achieve a positive outcome—growth and well-being of the child—the child's family or caregiver must be able to span the boundaries of the Vision Circle. The Vision Circle symbolizes a commitment to a working partnership among the local sectors of the community to assure improvement in the quality and structure of children's services. The Vision Circle is a metaphor for the process and structures to be developed and is perceived in the community as the new model of services.

Setting the Direction

The next step in the planning process involved setting the direction for developing the service system structure. A preliminary plan included identifying key goals, creating a statement of values, and defining ways to measure service outcomes. Three tasks emerged in this phase of the planning and system design process: 1) developing a preliminary regional service plan, 2) forming five service domain projects, and 3) forming integration teams.

1. Preliminary Regional Service Plan, June 1996. The steering committee produced a report, "Did We Hear You?" outlining the goals, objectives, and outcome indicators of the community working groups' submissions as well as other focus group and survey information representing 400 Calgary youth and consumers. This preliminary service plan addressed the interdependency

FIGURE 1 The Vision Circle

"It takes a whole village to raise a child"   African proverb

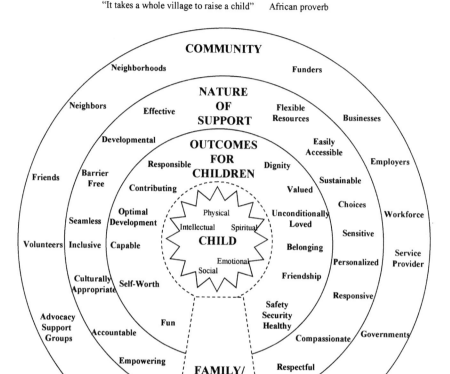

The outermost ring (the first ring) is our "village", our community. It contains the members of community who together, are responsible for using their resources and supports in ways described in the second ring, to help our children achieve the outcomes shown in the third ring.

The key to our children's development is their families/caregivers: their impact is evident in every ring of the vision circle.

At the very centre of the circle is the child.

Revised September 25, 1995, Calgary Rockyview Region.

between system participants and the need for organizational integration to ensure the fit identified in the Vision Circle. The importance of a logical and integrated interorganizational fit for the larger delivery system was emphasized.

Key Goals.   Based on the process to this point a preliminary service plan emerged with six key goals to serve the children and families in Calgary Rockyview:

1. Children, youth, and families are safe in their communities.
2. Comprehensive, integrated, safe, and individualized treatments, supports, and services for children with special needs and their families are developed and delivered.
3. Children, youth, and families are healthy.
4. Communities are involved in providing services for children, youth, and families.
5. Aboriginal peoples are involved in the delivery of services and resources for aboriginal children, youth, and families.
6. Rockyview regional child and family service authority's programs, services, and resources are integrated and effective.

The preliminary service plan recommended forming domain design groups for the delivery system design component.

Five Service Domain Groups, November 1996. Against the backdrop of the preliminary plans, visions, and goals the domain groups were formed with volunteers and nominees from the community to design the service strategies and plans for implementation. Five service planning domain groups were established: 1) day care, 2) family court and mediation for families, 3) protection of children and youth, 4) prevention of family violence, and 5) supporting children with special needs and their families.

Statutory and regulatory functions that are currently funded by the government, such as child protection investigations and the licensing of day care facilities as well as direct care services, such as placement programs for children, and women's shelters were to be integrated in the service delivery design. The domain committee reports were to be completed and submitted to the steering committee for the implementation plan. Five specific program delivery responsibilities or domains were to be transferred to each regional child and family service authority:

> Child welfare services—child protection, family services, children in care, and adoptions
>
> Services for special needs children and their families—lifestyle supports
>
> Family court and mediation services for families who are separating
>
> Prevention of family violence services, including women's shelters
>
> Day care services—licensing, monitoring, and consulting

Service Integration Teams, May 1997. Using the same process as that utilized for developing work groups, volunteers were solicited to form service integration teams charged with developing implementation guidelines for the five service domains. The work process for each of the service integration teams involved reviewing its service domain design and developing a plan for service integration that would result in a seamless array of services. The plans were submitted to the Regional Children and Family Services Steering Committee. A public forum was organized to present the implementation strategy to the community stakeholders for review and modifications. The revised integrated service plan was then submitted to the provincial government.

Developing Strategies for Implementation

Implementation strategies for the service domain outlined in the preliminary plan needed a policy framework. Legislation and standards provide the policy framework and the parameters within which local services are considered and will be implemented. Planning for implementation is in progress but some structures are in place.

Policy Framework. The provincial government passed the Child and Family Services Authorities Act (June 1997) enabling the seventeen regional authorities. An operating authority is now sanctioned in the Calgary Rockyview region and the legislation permits planning for and implementation of permanent structures and new roles and responsibilities. Under Alberta law, the provincial government is responsible for services for the safety, security, and well-being of children and families. This will not change under the new legislation. Under the Child and Family Services Authorities Act the provincial government has the following specific responsibilities:

Set objectives, policies, and standards for child and family services in Alberta

Allocate funding and other resources for the regional authorities

Monitor and assess the regional authorities in the carrying out of their responsibilities

As set out in the Child and Family Services Authorities Act the regional authority has the following specific responsibilities:

Assess needs, set priorities, plan, allocate resources, and manage the provision of services to children, families, and other community members in the region

Ensure that children and families have reasonable access to quality services

Ensure that provincial policies and standards are followed in the region

Monitor and assess the provision of child and family services

Work with other authorities, public and private bodies, and government to coordinate services for children and families (Office of the Minister, 1997)

The tasks will be implemented under the authority board and will work closely with communities in the region.

Structure.   With legislation in place, the regional child and family service authority was established in December 1997. The authority is charged with designing strategies and service delivery models that respond to the needs of local children, families, and communities. A selection panel representing stakeholders in the Calgary Rockyview region was formed by the Calgary Office of the Commissioner of Services for Children and Families. The selection panel reviewed applicants and recommended the selection of the fifteen members of the authority, now in place. A chief executive officer was hired to carry out the regional authority's policies and decisions, manage the day-to-day operations of the authority, and ensure that the regional structure runs effectively.

Business Plan.   The business plan will be the first task of the regional child and family services authority. It will build on the community's work to date and reflect how the service plan will be put into action as an operational service. Three elements are contained in the business plan:

1. *Service implementation planning.* The plan includes an idea of the communities who require service components. The scope of community-based services is linked to a community coordinating council, a community resource center and multiservice team structure. The plan addresses basic operational processes such as case management and teamwork,

2. *Identification of transition issues and options for implementation and phasing in services,*

3. *Operational planning.* The plan identifies key performance indicators, human resources and facility allocations, and contracted agencies to provide the designated services. The business plan includes the financial plan or budget request. Following approval of the business plan by the provincial government, the regional child and family services authority implements the integrated community service plan.

Funding Model.   The provincial government, through the Ministry of Family and Social Services, will provide funds on a block basis to each regional child and family services authority. The government will allocate to each authority a block of dollars to provide services to children and families in its region. The funding model will be reviewed in three years. It is not known what the exact financial allocation will be for each region, but a population-need-based model will be used for the calculations.

A consultation process set up by the government arrived at the funding model. The model's elements include relative risk, population need in general, higher need populations, and measurable indexes of service need. The population need model will be based on demographic factors including 1) the number of children aged 0–17 years in the region, weight 1; 2) the number of children from aboriginal people in the region, weight 6; 3) the number of children living in single parent families, weight 4; 4) the number of children from low-income families (based on nationally established indicators), weight 4.

Once funding is determined the envelope will be passed to the newly formed regional child and family authority to be allocated and implemented according to the four pillars of the initiative—integration of services, community-based services, improved aboriginal services, and early intervention initiatives—as well as fulfillment of the mandates transferred to the regional jurisdiction.

Funding may be adjusted under two circumstances: 1) base funding adjustment to factor in transportation, population density, and higher costs associated with providing services without economies of scale, and 2) secondary adjustments to compensate the authorities for other costs beyond their control. These costs would be identified and quantified in the authorities' business plans (Office of the Minister, 1997).

Funds will be distributed to each authority on a block basis (a lump sum to the region) with two exceptions. Envelope or set-aside funding (a specific amount for a specific area of service) will be provided for services and supports to children with disabilities and their families and for family violence prevention. These set-asides are to ensure that specific and equitable amounts of funding are allocated and used for the designated service areas. Administrative and operational costs will be funded in a different, single block. To ensure accountability, administrative and operational costs will be defined and identified separately in the business plan and then be tracked, monitored, and reported as distinct business items.

Providers of Service.   Funding for service provision will be done primarily through provincially developed contracts for annual and multiyear periods (Alberta Government, 1994). Services will be contracted on the basis of making available a certain kind of service to a set number of consumers, for example, six bed spaces for a community-based group home for youth. To a lesser extent, fee-for-service arrangements will continue to be used. These arrangements entail the provision of specific services to a client. Fee-for-service will be used when contracted blocks of services are full and additional services are needed on an emergency basis, or when contracted services cannot provide the needed services based on the specialized nature of the required service. In most instances standing offers of agreement or retainer types of agreements will be used with fee-for-service providers, setting standardized payment rates and specifying expectations about information restrictions and reporting.

Summary of the Process

The objectives of redesigning family and children's services is to respond to a demand for cost curtailment while addressing the need to improve the quality of care for children and families. Widespread community participation has been sought in the redesign process in order to ensure a publicly supported, high-quality child and family service authority. It is to the issue of quality that we now turn our attention.

QUALITY IN CHILD AND FAMILY SERVICES

"Quality" is a broadly defined conceptual framework for the new Calgary Rockyview regional system. Within the redesign initiative, quality is understood to consist of two components: the traditional outcome component and a process component. It is believed that a high-quality, local area service system demonstrates both efficient processes and effective outcomes.

The customary understanding of quality centers on outcomes. As such, quality refers to the impact of the services delivered by the system. The use of key performance indicators helps participants and stakeholders document progress toward desired outcomes. Key performance indicators and measures chosen must be appropriate, meaningful, and collected regularly. Data can then be used to solve problems, identify service gaps, and make program or service delivery adjustment. However, a shared language and common culture must exist for data to be collected and evaluation to be conducted. Therefore, a quality model of child and family services rests on data and measures that can be understood by those most affected—the stakeholders and participants.

The second meaning associated with quality focuses on interaction or process. Quality as a process centers on the decision-making mechanisms surrounding the service delivery system. Information and data need to be shared with all community stakeholders and participants, as well as serving as the foundation for funding and program direction. Quality as process is concerned with inclusion of stakeholders and community groups in the design, development, and ongoing evaluation of the new delivery system. In the redesign initiative, quality has been defined as stakeholder involvement in the processes of system design and service delivery.

At this time, neither performance standards nor process or outcome measures have been developed or adopted. These elements are in development. Community planning groups are forming local community coordinating councils to determine performance standards and measures. Community stakeholders are working to identify the set of expected results to be used as program-based benchmarks. Consideration is being given to establishing "best practice programs" and developing communication reports to serve as indicators of the changing individual or community environment. The regional child and family services authority and other participants are struggling with how to integrate assessment of performance indicators into routine evaluation and service processes.

The identification, selection, and implementation of benchmarks and key performance indicators are seen as vital steps in developing the quality monitoring system for Calgary Rockyview. Benchmarks will be developed to mark both system and client progress. They are intended to provide reference points and serve as a form of measurement in judging quality, value, and accountability. Key performance indicators will be instrumental in assessing the achievement of both process goals and outcome goals.

Quality as Planning Process of the Service Delivery System

The emphasis on quality as efficient processes began during the planning phase as the community planning groups assessed community needs, resources, and supports. As a quality indicator of efficiency, the community planning groups used participant feedback processes focused on each milestone. Extensive representation from various sectors and stakeholders was also solicited throughout the planning process and phases. For example, three town hall "gatherings" were held, with approximately 250 to 400 participants from public, private, and voluntary sectors of the community in attendance each time. At these meetings, the process involved opportunities for feedback and refinement of work from the various community planning groups. The town hall process was necessary to consolidate community strategies and to review the first milestones of work in the development of the preliminary children's service plan.

Four hundred additional participants and stakeholders were represented in the working groups, and a supplementary group of 200 adult and youth users of family and children's services participated in other one-time focus groups. Initiatives of special communities such as the aboriginal population and other culturally diverse populations were part of the inclusive community process.

The working groups and other community planning groups valued the town meetings as a mechanism for feedback to the Regional Children and Family Services Steering Committee on the process, ideas, interests, and even choice of wording in reports and planning documents. This process and resulting information formed the preliminary service plan for the implementation of services. Professionals may have experienced difficulty with the format and wording of documents—for example, the Vision Circle—but through this approach such products represented the consensus of the different community sectors.

Through the planning process, the community groups will determine whether the current and projected services relate to the goals, values, and objectives of the emerging system. Efficiency is to be measured by examining service delivery in four areas: 1) resource allocation, 2) service delivery, 3) sustained and systematic change environment, and 4) improved consumer and service outcomes.

Resource Allocation.   The process for planning and designing the service system focused on setting general planning directions as well as addressing both the number of services required and the scope of responsibilities for improving community-based services. This broad-based community planning strategy allows a reallocation of resources to develop a variety of services. Through the consensus process community members made decisions to reduce administrative costs while determining which of the existing programs would be maintained and which programs required revision. Maintaining a diverse choice of services is crucial to quality within a relevant community service model, and this result is considered most attainable when the community planning approach is inclusive.

Service Delivery.   The regional authority and community representatives are setting protocols to guide the authority and ensure that families who move from one region to another will have continuity in services. Regions will be able to share resources or purchase services from one another as needed; access to technical and other types of support from the government is available; and effective and efficient processes of administration are expected to be in place shortly.

Sustained and Systematic Change Environment.   Regular reporting of information to the regional authority, participants, the public, and other stakeholders of the service system is intended to promote an environment of constant improvement. Mechanisms will be established for communication and future joint planning between the authority and service providers. It is expected that both efficiency and effectiveness will be reported to the authority with at least the same frequency as used in the periodic reporting process for fiscal information. This will allow the directional change or self-correction that is rooted in the model's long-term vision.

Improved Consumer and Service Outcomes.   Direct communication with and accountability to the community is incorporated into the mandate of the regional authority. Presently, some services routinely evaluate their programs, but others will need to comply quickly with this component. Service organizations will need to strengthen their capabilities by integrating evaluation into ongoing components of service provision and to introduce periodic reflection and analysis into direct funding based on results. Consumers will have an opportunity to provide feedback through mechanisms yet to be determined.

Quality as Impact of Delivery System Services

The customary definition of quality focuses on the impact of delivered services. Quality implies improved functioning, improved practice customer satisfaction, service efficiency, and protection of consumer rights. In the Calgary Rockyview system, these quality indicators are still in development. The Alberta government is setting provincewide outcomes, and the regional authority, participants, and stakeholders are currently involved as a group in determining performance targets and measures of key performance indicators. The six key goals that were identified earlier in this chapter are standards that still need to be operationalized in the new model. These goals address the public, child, family, community, and service issues identified as driving the service redesign initiative. The six performance standards in their present form will be difficult to measure, and at this time some appear immeasurable. The impact of the system is to be determined by the following:

1. *Safety of children.* Services and families must lead to the improved well-being of children. Keeping families together is no substitute for children's developmental progress. Keeping families intact may or may not have a desirable outcome for children.

2. *Services and resources for special needs children and their families.* The population of high needs and special needs children and their families will participate in ensuring that necessary and sufficient services are provided for this group of individuals.

3. *Healthy development.* Child care environments need to emphasize health and other developmental needs of children. Health problems need to be recognized early and wherever possible prevented. Early identification services must be made available to address developmental delay, dental, growth, and mental health concerns. Child outcomes also need to take into account the child's interests, desires, and needs for adaptive developmental skills and education.

4. *Community-based services.* Staying in one's community is a desirable outcome for most individuals. Consumers who receive individualized service are involved in shaping or determining the kinds of services they will use, especially if these programs are in the neighborhoods where people live.

5. *Aboriginal specific resources and services.* The process of sustained and systematic service changes requires continuous inclusion of diverse community-based providers for child and family services. Aboriginal people will design specific resources and services for the aboriginal communities that will be delivered by aboriginal professionals and staff.

6. *Integrated and effective service.* A regional child and family services integration team will formally partner with other local authorities, including health, education, justice, social services, and municipalities. Other interdepartmental structures for integrated child and family services will also

be developed and will play a yet to be determined role in setting performance standards and establishing key performance indicators in this area. An integrated community council for children and family services, health, education, justice, social services, municipalities, and others, as a means of supporting overall community well-being, has been created.

REMAINING ISSUES: BUILDING AND BALANCING STRUCTURES AND PROCESSES

To date considerable progress has been made in the development of an integrated, managed social service system for Calgary Rockyview. However, many challenges remain to be addressed if the system is to fulfill its promise. Delicate interactions between and within the policy, managerial, and service domains will ultimately determine the success of the new model. Three challenges loom on the horizon and are possible constraints: motivation, staff secondment (reassignment) from the old system, and stakeholder preparation.

Maintaining Motivation

Much can be lost in implementation of strategies, including connection to and participation of the community, if motivation is lost. The extent to which motivation is maintained will depend on how well the first developmental stages of the model are implemented. The community's ongoing participation in planning and evaluating services and in the development of indicators will be the measure of success and a measure of maintained motivation. Feedback will show whether the processes are working.

Human Resources

Another challenge to implementation of the system involves the transition of staff to the redesigned system. In June 1997, the minister responsible for the redesign of services announced that in order to ensure that trained and qualified workers continue to deliver services under the new community-based system, current Family and Social Service staff would be seconded or loaned to the seventeen regional authorities. The seconded staff will take their direction from each of the regional authorities. The government and the Calgary Rockyview community will have to determine how the government employees will be integrated into the service delivery system. The key will be to engage the community in resolving this issue. Managing a well-educated, highly skilled, and expensive labor force requires community agencies and organizations to pay particular attention to hiring, training, and determining which staff will be retained. The "inherited" staff must be given an opportunity to develop new roles and competencies. Compensation strategies must also support the organization's overall objective to ensure a coordinated, focused approach by the workforce. As for the government staff, there will be a need to address the transition from government employment to reshaping a new role in various programs and services.

Stakeholder Preparation

Professionals, nonprofessionals, other stakeholders, and service providers will need to redefine their roles as partners with the informal community networks and other sectors. The professional staff of the government will need to see themselves as bringing technical expertise to children, families, and community. This expertise is strongly valued within the community, but it is seen as being different from professionally, governmentally controlled services. Some Calgary Rockyview organizations may need to make considerable changes in their programs in terms of the structure, content, and process of service management, including the locality or site for program delivery. All service providers will have to form new alliances and partnerships because they must engage in collaborative relationships across service sectors for the first time. Change in professional staff practice, both in terms of policy and management, may be considered a barometer of the change initiative's success as the system moves toward integration.

COMMON PURPOSE INTO THE FUTURE

The Calgary Rockyview region children's services network is undergoing a change in relationships and roles with the children, families, and communities they serve. The new structure is being driven by the need to form community partnerships that serve the interests and needs of localities as well as emphasize practice that reduces risks of common problems. The partnerships articulate a common purpose. During the past two years, the transition has involved a planning and redesign process. Nearly 12,000 Albertans have volunteered their time, energy, and knowledge to plan a more efficient and effective delivery system. The operation of the service delivery system is inextricably linked to a set of core values or principles that reflect sensitivity to community, social and cultural diversity, and flexibility. Quality is defined as the continuous involvement of stakeholders in a community-based service system and in improvements of the system. It is more than compliance activities. Quality is about establishing processes to review how both the process and services affect the consumers or services.

Community participation in the design of children's services introduces variation in services at the local level and transforms the child-serving system. A common and comprehensive purpose to managing resources and services that blends public and private sector entities is desired. The outcome of this program implementation process is still in the future. It is a process with many unknowns. If the redesigned service system is to succeed, common purpose and shared responsibility must be maintained between the regional child and families service authority and the community. Ongoing training, development, and preparation with all stakeholders is essential as this community moves toward the next developmental stage. At this point, the change initiative has succeeded in mobilizing and stimulating community resources and participants, but the implementation phase will present new challenges.

REFERENCES

Alberta Children's Advocate. (1993). *In need of protection: Children and youth in Alberta. Child welfare review.* Edmonton, AB: Department of Family and Social Services.

Alberta Commissioner of Services for Children and Families. (1995, May). *Service planning handbook.* Edmonton, AB: Department of Family and Social Services.

Alberta Commissioner of Services for Children and Families. (1997, November). Recommended model for the distribution of provincial funding for Child and Family Services Funding Model Committee. Edmonton, AB: Author.

Alberta Family and Social Services. (1994). *Focus on Children.* Edmonton, AB: Queens Printer.

Alberta Government. (1994, Spring). *Performance management.* Connexus: Queens Printer.

Calgary Rockyview Draft Preliminary Service Plan. (1996). *Did we hear you? Work in progress.* Calgary, AB: Commissioner's Office of Children's Services.

Canada West Foundation. (1996). Expenditures for Alberta children and youth. Calgary, AB: Author.

Mackenzie, B. (1991). Decentralization in Winnipeg: Assessing the effects of community based child welfare services. *Canadian Review of Social Policy, 27,* 57–66.

Ministry of Supply and Services. (1994). *Child welfare in Canada: The role of provincial and territorial authorities in cases of child abuse.* Ottawa: Health Canada, Federal Provincial Working Group on Child and Family Services Information.

Office of the Minister Responsible for Children's Services. (1997, November). *Final recommendations of Funding Model Committee for Child and Family Services.* Alberta Minister Without Portfolio. Edmonton, AB: Author.

Rothery, M., Gallup, J., Tillman, G., & Allard, H. (1995). Local governance of child welfare services in Alberta. *Child Welfare, 74*(3), 587–603.

Thomlison, R. J. (1984). *Case management review. Northwest Region, Department of Social Services and Community Health.* Unpublished report, University of Calgary, Faculty of Social Work.

U.S. Department of Health and Human Services. (1996, June 11). *HHS invests in America's children* [Press Release].http://www.os.dhhs.gov/news/press/960611.html.

Weisman, M. (1994, July). When parents are not in the best interests of the child: "Family preservation" has become child-welfare dogma—but some children need institutional care. *Atlantic Monthly,* pp. 43–44, 46–47, 50-54, 56–60, 62–63.

Weithorn, L. (188). Mental hospitalization of troublesome youth: An analysis of skyrocketing admission rates. *Standard Law Review, 40,* 663-738.

Werrbach, G. B. (1992). A study of home-based services for families of adolescents. *Child and Adolescent Social Work Journal, 9,* 505-523.

PART TWO

The Service Delivery System

The four case studies that follow document the impact of managed care on the delivery systems of human service organizations. These business cases describe the nature of contemporary human service work in classic social work agencies. Two cases discuss experiences in family service agencies. One case reports on the experience of a child welfare agency. One case reports on the experience of a mental health agencies.

The cases here reveal three major themes. First, the service delivery system operates in a dynamic, ever changing environment. Although change has always existed for human service organizations, the nature of change has been transformed. The time frame of environmental change has shortened. The participants or key actors involved have multiplied exponentially. Together these facets of change force human service organizations to attend constantly to their operational environments.

Second, the context of human service work has changed fundamentally from stable to unstable. Shifts in the operating environment have become so unpredictable that the human service organization must be both vigilant and prepared to respond quickly. The context has also become more business oriented, as discussed in part 1. Beyond caring for those in need, human service organizations must now demonstrate implementation of sound business practices. This new requirement is partly due to the growing impact of market forces on human services. Barriers that prevented for-profit organization from competing for government human service contracts have fallen. Nonprofit human service organizations are now expected not only to operate but to *compete* effectively. With the growth of the service economy, for-profit service organizations have entered into provision of human services for even the most vulnerable populations.

Third is the new role for the human administrator. The skill set and preparation of the new human service administrator must be radically different from those in previous generations. More than in the past, business acumen and the concomitant skills must accompany an understanding of the human services. The new human service administrator must know, understand, and be able to communicate the "product line" or aspect of the social work agency and, at the same time, drive, direct, and determine the business operation of the organization. These skill sets may seem to be mutually exclusive. However, if human service organizations cannot do well while doing good, they will fail in this new environment.

Each of the four cases depicts all these themes, but with greater emphasis on one or another. In chapter 6 Buescher and Wernet describe the dynamic intraorganizational environment created by managed care. The case report on the evolution of the service operations and the organizational planning of a family service agency and the dismantling of the organization's managed care operation.

In chapter 7 Sidwell discusses the changes that have influenced the operational strategies and thinking of an administrative officer within a family service agency. He describes an innovative and entrepreneurial joint venture, in which a wholly owned, for-profit subsidiary was created.

Barker and Wernet describe in chapter 8 the evolution of a traditional child treatment center. This case describes a series of options explored in maintaining the organization's vitality in the face of uncertainty. The case demonstrates the impact of a managed care system on the strategic development of a children's service agency.

In chapter 9 Christian-Michaels, Noll, and Wernet present a case study of a mental health service embedded within a public health department. They describe the impact of complex interinstitutional forces, expectations, and professional practices on the restructuring of a quasi-public mental health service. The authors examine the interplay of devolution and privatization and the manager's use of these issues to refine the organization's focus and dedication to meeting the needs of the severely and profoundly mentally ill.

Taken together, these four cases depict innovators in and early adopters of managed care in human service organizations. The first two cases focus on leading-edge organizations. They were innovative in addressing and incorporating a new approach—managed care—into their operations. True to form, these organizations have also abandoned this arena of business—first in, first out. They and their administrators have experienced both the opportunities and the costs associated with the leading edge of change.

The last two cases report on the experiences of early adopters of managed care. These organizations remained in the mainstream of human service operations. Unlike the innovators, these early adopters modified components of existing operations in order to respond to the demands of managed care. They represent the beginnings of mainstream response to managed care through modification and accommodation rather than innovation and transformation. Together these four cases reveal the options for organizational change.

CHAPTER 6

Managed PsychCare

Kathleen E. Buescher

President and Chief Executive Officer,
Provident Counseling, Inc., Saint Louis

Stephen P. Wernet

Professor, School of Social Service,
Saint Louis University

The following is the story of Provident Counseling's venture into behavioral health care and the development, and eventual demise, of its behavioral health program, Managed PsychCare. Provident Counseling is a tax-exempt, 501(c)3, family service agency in Saint Louis, Missouri, whose mission is "to further the well-being of individuals, families and communities by managing and delivering high quality mental and behavioral health care services, including counseling, training and education, advocacy, case management, referral, prevention services, research and community outreach" (Board of Directors, May 1994). Programs are delivered by a multidisciplinary staff composed of caseworkers, counselors, nurses, psychiatrists, psychologists, and social workers. Annually, more than 20,000 families receive services through the agency's numerous service locations throughout the eight-county metropolitan Saint Louis area.

During the 1970s, two developments occurred that helped prepare Provident Counseling for managed care. First, the board and staff became interested

The first author thanks several persons for help in the preparation of this case study: Robert Frank, Bruce Buckland, and Einar Ross, all former members of Provident's board of directors; Barbara Buenemann, vice president and chief operating officer, United Healthcare of the Midwest; Phil Crause, executive vice president, Managed PsychCare, Provident Counseling; Don Cuvo, executive director, City of St. Louis Mental Health Board of Trustees; Dianne Kimbro, quality assurance specialist, United Behavioral Health; and Barbara Scheiper-Latal, president, Life Designs.

in serving the needs of people in industry. Thus the agency began to offer employee assistance services to employers. Second, counseling services became reimbursable from insurance companies. The agency had its first contract with Blue Cross/Blue Shield of Missouri for mental health counseling services to local United Auto Workers (UAW) members. This led to similar arrangement with other insurance companies. Staff auditing for the appropriateness of care and treatment planning was also provided within these arrangements. Little did we realize that these were the first steps toward managed care.

INCUBATION PERIOD, 1979–1987

Between 1979 and 1987, Provident expanded its partnership programs with industry. Agency skills and talents were matched with the needs of business. This expansion occurred through two programs, employee assistance and customer service, and professional accreditation.

Employee Assistance Program

In the later 1970s the idea of offering an employee assistance program (EAP) was germinating among the board and the staff. This development was in response to a local engineering firm's request for service provision to its employees. The EAP offered short-term counseling (usually three to six sessions annually) to employees of the contracting company and their dependents. Supervisors also used the EAP as a resource for an employee whose job performance appeared to be affected by a personal problem. In the beginning, the EAP services were targeted to identify and assist the alcoholic employee.

Support from a foundation and the United Way was secured to cover start-up costs for the EAP. Unlike many other EAPs, staff were not recovering alcoholics. Rather they were highly trained professionals with advanced degrees.

Formidable competition developed in the EAP marketplace. A locally based, for-profit EAP objected to Provident's foray into this arena. Attempts were made both to discredit the agency and to stop it from providing EAP services. It was suggested to employers that Provident's facilities were "no better than welfare offices." The red flag of "unfair competition" was also waved by the opposing company.

Provident was one of the family service agencies in the country to provide EAP services. The organization was perceived as a pioneer even though there was great resistance to viewing alcoholism as a primary problem.

Customer Assistance Program

In 1986, the local electric utility company decided to develop a customer assistance program. Through research, the utility company learned that the cause of sudden, unexpected payment difficulties of formerly good-paying customers was some type of personal or family crisis such as unemployment, divorce or separation, illness, or disability. In deciding to deliver a remedial service program, the company realized it needed to go outside itself. Provident was the successful bidder for the service contract. Through this program, the agency had a new opportunity to work closely with business and industry. Instead of providing services to a company's employees, the agency was working directly with the company's customers.

External Professional Accreditation

Insurance companies and other third-party purchasers of services were increasingly asking for professional licensure for its mental health service providers. Simultaneously, and several years after the start of Provident's EAP services, the staff concluded that stronger identification with the health care industry would benefit the agency. Subsequently, in 1982, the agency sought and obtained accreditation from the Joint Commission on the Accreditation of Healthcare Organizations. This accreditation was seen as an enhancement of the organization's standards. Joint Commission accreditation was, and continues to be, an indicator that an organization met the highest standards of operation and service of the health care field. Accreditation also meant that the professional staff met credentialing and privileging criteria, a substitute for, the as yet unavailable, professional licensure. This accreditation confirmed Provident's shift in organizational identity from social service agency to health care provider and solidified its identification with the health care industry.

DEVELOPMENT AND OPERATION OF MANAGED PSYCHCARE, 1987–1998

A timeline of the history of Managed PsychCare is depicted in table 1. The narrative that follows explains the events that occurred surrounding the development, operation, and eventual demise of Managed PsychCare.

Opportunity

In 1987 a major nationwide insurance company became dissatisfied with the payouts on its psychiatric and substance abuse benefits. Inpatient care was being used when a less intense level of care could have been as, or more, effective. Premiums were increasing at a rate high enough to make the company's policies noncompetitive. Following a study of its alternatives, the company identified three options: 1) purchase a behavioral health provider group, 2) reduce psychiatric and substance abuse benefits, or 3) subcontract psychiatric and substance abuse services using "risk-based" arrangements. The company chose the last option and pilot tested the new model in the Saint Louis region.

TABLE 1   History of Managed PsychCare

1987–1995	Managed PsychCare contracts with MetLife
July 1, 1994	Managed PsychCare takes over capitated Network Operations in Kansas City Network
January 1, 1995	MetLife and Travelers merge their health care divisions to form MetraHealth Corporation
August 1, 1995	Managed PsychCare takes over claims administration from MetraHealth Corporation
October 1, 1995	MetraHealth is acquired by United HealthCare
July 1, 1996	United Healthcare takes over Kansas City business; Managed PsychCare no longer serves the Kansas City market
July 1996	United HealthCare is required to sell MetraHealth HOMO business in the Saint Louis market but keeps other product lines of MetraHealth
	Principle Health Care acquires HMO business product line from United HealthCare
January 1, 1997–March 31, 1998	Managed PsychCare provides capitated services for Principal Health care members through its subsidiary, Principal Behavioral HealthCare
October 1, 1997	Principal HealthCare sells its wholly owned behavioral health company, Principle Behavioral Health Care to American Psych Systems
January 1, 1998	Principal Health Care is acquired by Coventry Health
April 1, 1998	Provident Counseling establishes a provider contract with American Psych Systems on a case rate basis.

In Saint Louis, the insurance company was a partner with several hospitals, a medical school, and a physician group practice in a health maintenance organization (HMO). The insurance company bought out the other partners and decided to subcontract psychiatric and substance abuse services to an independent provider group. The contract was to be risk based; that is, it was structured as a carved-out model with financial risks to be assumed by the contractee.

The HMO wanted a provider to assume responsibility for the full scope of psychiatric and substance abuse services, including inpatient, partial hospitalization, intensive outpatient, and outpatient services. The HMO was unable at that time to provide full and complete information about the prior utilization of psychiatric and substance abuse benefits from which good rates could be determined. This was not unusual in 1987. The data were either not maintained or not collected in useful ways. Few HMOs, insurance companies, or self-insured employers fully understood the utilization of psychiatric and substance abuse benefits by their enrollees. However, they did know that as a bundle, psychiatric and substance abuse services were extremely expensive.

In March 1987 Provident was invited to bid on the carved-out contract. The magnitude of the opportunities such a relationship could bring to the agency was quite clear. The bid required the successful applicant to assume responsibility for client care along with the financial risk for a full range of services. Provident had never before assumed professional or financial responsibility for the delivery or management of inpatient services. To be successful the agency would require new skill sets:

Ability to assess the level of care needed by a client

Ability to develop criteria for admission, continued stay, and discharge from the hospital

Ability to negotiate rates and services with hospitals and partial hospitalization program providers

In spring 1987 the board of directors met to discuss the proposal. Some board members urged caution about accepting the financial risk, especially for services the agency was unaccustomed to managing. Concerns were raised about insurance and liability. Would the agency be considered an insurer if it assumed these risks? Would the state want to regulate the agency as if it was an HMO? What would this program do to professional liability costs? Would a big claim threaten the financial solvency of the agency?

Board members saw several potential benefits to entering a managed care contract. A portion of the agency's fixed operating expenses could be spread over these new services. There was potential for increased visibility for Provident in the employer community. Any surplus revenues earned on this contract could be infused into agency services for low-income, uninsured clients. It was an opportunity to further broaden and diversify the agency's fiscal base and financial security thereby making it better able to withstand the vagaries of any particular funding source.

There was certain appeal to adding to Provident's organizational capabilities while doing more with its staff talent. Unlike EAP services, in which great pains are taken to avoid the appearance of "feathering one's own nest," there is a great advantage to keeping outpatient services under the organization's umbrella. Control of service utilization and their related costs is the foundation of a managed care approach. If Provident could assure high-quality service and control both utilization and cost by referring to its own staff, then the organization had a good chance of being able to deliver services within the financial constraints of the contract. In a managed care contract, there is no incentive to make unnecessary referrals even within your own organization. There is no benefit to overutilizing services because costs increase unnecessarily.

One individual was instrumental in helping to allay the fears of his peers on the board of directors. He was looked to for assurance and confidence that Provident was capable of delivering on such a contract. This individual was a recently retired hospital administrator who had served for twenty years as the president of the largest, most prestigious hospital in Saint Louis. He was a highly regarded professional who was valued for his expertise and opinions. He helped the staff think through and construct its contract proposal. Coincidentally, he sat on the board of the HMO but steadfastly maintained an arm's length distance from all decision-making processes and decision votes in both organizations.

Provident brought several advantages to the negotiating table. HMO enrollees would have convenient access to outpatient services because of Provident's multiple service delivery sites across the metropolitan area. Provident had met the health care industry's highest standards with its accreditation by the Joint Commission. The agency enjoyed a positive reputation in the community and was known for high-quality outpatient services. The agency's standing within the medical and psychiatric community was strong, thereby avoiding physician resistance to using Provident as an outpatient provider. It was later learned that Provident was the lead contender, and the standard against which other bidders were judged, because of both its numerous and dispersed area offices and its Joint Commission accreditation.

At their meeting on June 17, 1987, the executive committee empowered to act on behalf of the board voted to enter into a carved-out contract with the HMO, but only for outpatient services. Because of both incomplete data and its inexperience with services other than outpatient, Provident was reluctant to assume the full range of services until an experience level could be determined. When it had more experience managing care and utilization figures could be more accurately estimated, Provident would consider assuming responsibility for the full range of services.

The financial arrangements with the HMO were developed as a capitated rate. This was a negotiated dollar figure applied to the enrollment level of the group on a monthly basis (rate × number of enrollees each month). The rate was projected to cover all expenses for managing and delivering psychiatric and substance abuse services to the enrolled population.

First Contract: Managed PsychCare Is Born

Managed PsycheCare (initially called Care Management) was established to deliver services effective July 1, 1987. Its initial purpose was to manage all outpatient psychiatric and substance abuse care. Three new staff members were hired: a director and a therapist, both of whom were masters'-level-prepared psychiatric nurses, and a secretary. The initial plan was for Managed PsychCare to handle all outpatient services itself. Because the demand quickly outstripped Managed PsychCare's ability to handle it, and clients needed convenient geographic access, the substantial resources of the agency's counseling staff were soon tapped.

The financial pressure the HMO had experienced due to excess inpatient utilization did not disappear with the outsourcing of outpatient services. Even though the utilization figures for inpatient services were still not fully available, renegotiation of the contract began in September for a January 1, 1998, start date. After several months of work, the board approved the new contract in November 1987.

On January 1, 1988, Managed PsychCare assumed responsibility for managing the full scope of behavioral health care services. Managed Psych-Care staff admitted clients to care and managed the services while the agency's counseling staff delivered the care. Managed PsychCare staff served as utilization reviewers, assessing medical necessity of requested services, authorizing admission, and determining both its intensity and duration. The agency's medical director monitored inpatient care. Overnight and weekend response was contracted out to a hospital-based group.

Within weeks of start-up, service utilization was dramatically above estimates. By the end of February inpatient utilization was three times higher than projected. Several factors contributed to these high utilization rates. The group handling overnight and weekend response was placing individuals into, rather than diverting them from, inpatient facilities. Managed PsychCare was referring to other psychiatrists in the community because its medical director was unable to handle the load of referrals generated by the program. These phenomena made control of utilization and quality more difficult than originally anticipated in the proposal.

The final issue of concern was the new contract's capitated rate. It was too low given the actual utilization being experienced. Both parties understood that the figures used to compute the original rate were suspect. Because both parties had invested heavily in the success of this new venture, neither wanted it to fail. Therefore, the HMO was willing to renegotiate the rate as the agency made other, internal changes to gain better control of utilization.

Several internal changes were completed as part of the contract renegotiations. The program's after-hours coverage was assumed by Managed PsycheCare. A third psychiatric nurse who had both hospital and insurance industry experience was hired to oversee utilization management for the program. A new medical director, whose approach was more "managed care friendly," was hired. He viewed outpatient care as a viable alternative to hospitalization. The new medical director was associated with a psychiatric group practice that had offices throughout the community, on which Managed PsychCare could draw.

Expansion of Managed PsychCare

Managed PsychCare's original staffing design started to change almost immediately. Outpatient services were provided by Provident counselors.

Managed PsychCare staff focused on utilization review. Later, a provider relations staff person and a second secretary were hired.

Managed PsychCare developed two models of service delivery: a staff model in which Provident therapists served as an internal preferred provider organization (PPO) and a network model in which Managed PsychCare contracted with vendors in the community for the work that Provident staff could not provide, such as inpatient, intensive outpatient, partial hospitalization, and overflow outpatient services. In the beginning, all Provident therapists were referred Managed PsychCare cases. Managed PsychCare also used all the hospitals and other providers who had contracts with the HMO and its network of external providers. Over time, participants in both models were reduced. The internal PPO was constricted to those clinicians interested in doing managed care work who had received specialized training. The external network was constricted to those institutions most interested in having managed care business and with whom the best working relationships had been developed.

In 1994, two additional part-time utilization managers were hired to handle services in Kansas City. The Managed PsychCare director's position was consolidated with the EAP director's position, reporting directly to the chief operating officer and in a job grade comparable to other program directors (see figure 1). With Managed PsychCare's expansion into the Kansas City market, a PPO relationship was established with Heart of America Family Services. Although they were part of Managed PsychCare's network of service providers in Kansas City, Heart of America operated as a staff model PPO for the majority of outpatient services required by the HMO's enrollees.

Financial Arrangements with the HMO.   The contract included a holdback that the HMO would use to pay hospital, physician, and "outside therapists" claims. Network providers contracting with Managed PsychCare would submit their claims directly to the HMO. The portion of the capitated contract that Provident received each month covered the expenses for both managing care and providing outpatient services by Provident's staff model internal PPO.

At the annual contract renewal date, Provident and the HMO attempted to calculate a breakeven figure to cover what was expected to be needed to pay hospital and physician costs. The HMO held back an amount from the capitation rate to pay these claims. The holdback amount was adjusted based on claims experience. Because there always were claims incurred but not reported, it was nearly impossible to reconcile precisely on the holdback amount due Provident.

The holdback amount provided a cushion in the event of a catastrophic claim. This was a concern when analyzing the risk-based contract. Reinsuring against such a risk was considered but discarded due to the prohibitive cost. Rather, the agency's limits on professional liability and directors and officers insurance were raised to accommodate the increased risk.

FIGURE 1   Chart of Organization

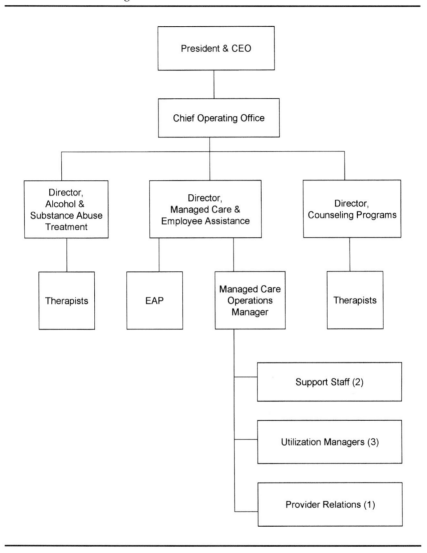

In 1994, which saw the apex of Managed PsychCare's operation, its capitation revenue was nearly $2 million. Of that, two-thirds was set aside to pay for treatment services of hospital care, physician services, and outpatient treatment for covered members. Staff salaries and benefits made up 16% of the budget, with operating expenses at 5%. These operating expenses do not include costs for enhanced management information services, which were substantial.

In mid-1994, the full-risk, capitated service contract expanded to include the Kansas City site as well as the processing and payment of claims management on the entire contract, thereby eliminating the holdback practice. This arrangement for the full capitation amount gave Provident better control over service claims authorization and payment.

Managed PsychCare had a surplus at the end of each operating year. Provident used these funds to subsidize its services to low-income, uninsured counseling clients and to cover general operating expenses. Managed Psych-Care was an important source of financial support to the total agency. In addition to its surplus, Managed PsychCare purchased services from the counseling program at a level to nine full-time therapists, or 20% of the counseling staff.

Risk-Based Contracts.   In addition to managing care, Provident also managed the cost of the care. Provident and the HMO arrived at a capitated rate for which Provident believed it could assume the financial risk of managing the cost of care. The rate was based on the number of members of the enrolled group, the expected utilization of all services, and the cost of providing those services. Expected utilization rates were based on the program's experiences and calculated in a "days per thousand" members formula. (The formula calculates the number of days of inpatient care or partial hospitalization services provided to a group of HMO members over a period of time, usually a month or a year. The resulting number is then divided by the total number of members and multiplied by 1,000.)

By establishing a capitated rate with Provident, the HMO contained its own psychiatric and substance abuse costs and incited Provident to manage this part of the health care benefit. If service utilization and its associated costs could be managed within the dollars provided through the capitated rate, Provident stood to earn a surplus. On the other hand, should utilization be higher than expected, or the costs of providing the care greater than planned, the agency was at risk of losing money.

Managed PsychCare and three types of contracts with the HMO and one type of contract with other behavioral health care companies: The first contract with the HMO was risk based with a capitated rate. It covered 35,000 to 40,000 enrollees in Missouri, Kansas, and Illinois. The HMO carved out its psychiatric and substance abuse services from its other medical benefits and contracted them to Provident's Managed PsychCare program.

The second HMO contract was for point of service. It was capitated but did not carry financial risk. Managed PsychCare provided gatekeeping services through its utilization management staff but did not assume any financial responsibility for the treatment service provided. Enrollees contacted Managed PsychCare for treatment authorization and referral to a Managed PsychCare network provider. If Managed PsychCare referred a point-of-service client to Provident's counseling program for outpatient care, the agency collected a client copayment and billed the HMO directly for a fee for service. Forty thousand enrollees were covered by this contract.

The third HMO contract was for services to a small number of HMO members living in out-of-state areas where there were no established provider networks managed by Managed PsychCare. Fewer than 3,000 enrollees were covered with this plan. Managed PsychCare was paid on a capitated basis for utilization management services but assumed no financial risk for the treatment. When the psychiatric or substance abuse services were requested by these members, Managed PsychCare identified providers in the nonnetwork areas and negotiated service arrangements and reimbursement rates for treatment.

Finally, Provident had a number of contracts with other behavioral health care companies to provide outpatient services to their enrollees on a preestablished, fee-for-service basis. Provident was part of the companies' provider panels. There were a few surprises with this type of contract. Some contracts had arrangements in which Provident's individual therapists were declared the preferred provider; if the clinician left Provident, they took provider status with them to a new agency or private practice. Staff were added to handle what was expected to be a large number of referrals from a company, only to have the company expand its own geographic coverage rather than refer to the agency.

Utilization Experience

At the time Provident responded to the HMO's request for a full-risk, capitated contract, the HMO did not have complete utilization information on which Provident could base its projections. A target was established of 43 days per 1,000 for inpatient services and 21 days per 1,000 for both partial hospitalization and intensive outpatient program services. Table 2 illustrates Managed PsychCare's experience. In eight of the ten years, the agency met or exceeded its utilization targets for inpatient services, while it met or exceeded its target for partial hospitalization and intensive outpatient services in only six years of operation.

Several factors influenced utilization levels:

1. Utilization managers assured that the intensity (level of care required) and duration (length of time, number of sessions, or number of days) of care were within reasonable limits for the diagnosis. Inpatient care, the most intense level of care, was used for stabilizing a client. Once stabilized, the client's level of care was "stepped down" to partial hospitalization and outpatient services.

2. The internal PPO network was constricted. Strict guidelines for provider credentialing were established by the HMO. The internal PPO network was then limited to therapists working full time at Provident who met the credentialing criteria and were interested in working with managed care cases.

TABLE 2   Utilization Information for Managed PsychCare

Year	Inpatient Days per 1,000	Partial & Intensive Outpatient Days per 1,000
1988	48.3	24.9
1989	34.1	14.6
1990	43.6	26.3
1991	32.7	21.1
1992	35.6	21.1
1993	19.0	13.0
1994	24.8	17.7
1995	17.7	15.3
1996	13.4	11.3
1997	17.8	14.3

3. The network of provider hospitals was reduced. In the beginning, Managed PsychCare used every hospital that had a contract with the HMO. Because this arrangement was terribly unwieldy, the network was reduced to six hospitals. After several year's experience, the Managed PsychCare provider hospital network was reduced to those two facilities with which the best working relationships had been established. These hospitals were found to consistently apply Managed PsychCare's assessment model, thereby eliminating the need for Managed PsychCare on-call staff to visit the hospital to conduct on-site assessment.

4. The use of partial hospitalization and intensive outpatient services was increased. These were alternatives to more costly inpatient care, which was limited to use for medical stabilization.

Demise of Managed PsychCare

Between 1994 and 1998, the behavioral health care marketplace experienced unprecedented change and turmoil. In Saint Louis in particular, there were consolidations and increased competition. These events forced Managed PsychCare and Provident to reevaluate this work in the managed behavioral health care marketplace. This review stimulated numerous organizational changes. In particular, these external changes led to the eventual closure of Managed PsychCare. Corporate consolidations, declining capitation rates, and increased assignment of risk to the provider coalesced to help drive Provident out of the managed care marketplace. However, this departure occurred later rather than earlier. Managed PsychCare's prolonged survival can be attributed to several strategies and tactics that are part of the organization's culture.

Marketplace Changes.   The behavioral health care marketplace has experienced consolidation and centralization of inordinate proportions during the past four years. In 1995 and 1996, three mergers and acquisitions occurred that affected Provident's managed care operation. In early 1995, the HMO with which Provident contracted was merged with the health care line of another insurer. Before the relationship could be solidified, the newly merged company was acquired by yet a third national HMO in mid-1995. Two of these three HMOs had wholly owned behavioral health subsidiaries. This newly created health care entity owned more than 50% of the HMO market share in Saint Louis. The Missouri Department of Insurance required this new entity to divest itself of the Saint Louis portion of the acquired company. In July 1996, a national insurer with a behavioral health subsidiary brought the divested business. Less than two years later, the health and behavioral health entities of this company had each been separately sold.

This market consolidation through mergers and acquisitions had a mixed effect on behavioral health care providers. In 1995, these consolidations had the unanticipated effect of returning decision making to the local level. Operational decisions were returned to the companies' local managers. This was an advantage to Provident because of its long-standing relationships with various operational managers. As the local managers advanced up the corporate operational ladders, they retained their preference for local decision making. However, in 1997 as the marketplace consolidated further with outside purchases of local companies, locally connected managers were either replaced or subsumed, and decision making and control were removed and centralized into the larger corporate operations. Therefore, although consolidation occurred in the marketplace, its negative impact on local operations like Provident's was not felt until much later than expected, or anticipated, by providers.

Another outcome of these mergers was increased competition in the marketplace. This competition took several forms. The numbers of bidders for provider contracts increased. This bidder increase was exacerbated by the reduction in the number of behavioral health care purchasers due to acquisitions and mergers. Another factor in increased competition was the existence of behavioral health care provider arms within the purchasers of other providers. In some circumstances, these factors led to increased price competition through either bidding wars or suppression of reimbursement rates. Managed PsychCare's rates dropped from a high of $4 per member per month in 1994 to a low of $2.35 per member per month in 1997, which was that portion of the rate designated by the subsidiary for treatment services and utilization management. In 1994, Provident was the behavioral health care contractor. By 1997, it was solely a subcontractor to the insurer's behavioral health care subsidiary.

The final marketplace change was targeted reductions. During this time period, managed care companies were generally attempting to achieve cost savings and maintain competitive rates for purchasers. These goals were reached in large part by reducing benefit packages, reimbursements, and margins. Behavioral health care benefits in particular were targeted for reductions in this push for cost savings.

Organizational Changes.   As a result of these marketplace changes, Provident Counseling had to implement numerous structural changes. These responses were accommodations not only to the three years of financial reductions associated with lost revenues in Managed PsychCare but to the decade-long general pattern of declining resources for human services.

Restructuring occurred in two waves. The first change took place in 1996. Responsibility for fiscal and operational monitoring was delegated to management staff. As part of this change, several offices were downsized, and some clinical and administrative staff were laid off. The second wave of restructuring was delayed from 1997 until 1998. A deficit budget was adopted for this one year. Unfortunately, in January 1998 Provident again downsized due to both the deficit and the loss of Managed PsychCare contracts. Again, some staff was laid off, and an expensive office center was closed. As additional consolidation, a layer of managers was eliminated from the organizational structure. As a result of both restructurings, one location was closed, three were downsized, and twenty-four staff positions were eliminated, which included six management positions.

IMPACT OF MANAGED CARE ON PROVIDENT COUNSELING

The impact of managed care on Provident has been substantial. It has influenced all aspects of the organization, its operation, and its staff. This section will discuss managed care's influence on the clinical staff, the treatment approach of the staff and agency, organizational structure, client population, performance and outcome assessments, and management and administrative operations.

Clinical Staff and Treatment Approach

The first few years of managed care services were difficult for Provident's counseling staff. Even today, there is no unanimity among the clinical staff that venturing into managed care services was a good idea.

As Managed PsychCare got underway, the plan was to provide outpatient treatment services through a resident clinical staff. Provident had successfully operated its EAP with its own internal staff, so it seemed logical to use the same design with Managed PsychCare. However, the high demand for outpatient services, the advantages of geographic accessibility, and the desire to use an experienced, competent staff soon made it inevitable that Provident's counseling staff should deliver Managed PsychCare's outpatient services.

Counseling staff was in the midst of a paradigm shift for which the agency and the environment had inadequately prepared them. Therapists were trying to fit their traditional model of client treatment into the new managed care model—with frustrating results. Case assignments were made to individual therapists at the agency's several counseling centers. Therapists were asked to provide services within a shorter, more focused time frame, that is, using between ten and twenty sessions. Therapists were asked routinely by Managed PsychCare's managers about treatment goals and progress toward them. Treatment had to be authorized every three or four sessions.

Therapists were bumping up against the concept of medical necessity. Insurance companies and self-insured employers were shifting away from open-ended psychiatric and substance abuse benefits. No longer did payers believe it was appropriate to reimburse for long-term talk therapy. For medical insurance to pay, the member's problem had to be one that met a screening for medical necessity.

Although they had experience providing services to some national and regional behavioral health care vendors, staff sometimes resisted the control and direction exerted by utilization reviewers associated with these vendors. Clinical staff often resented the requirement that service be authorized and bristled when held to limits on duration of treatment. Utilization review was perceived as antithetical to high-quality clinical practice and professional clinical decision making.

The new brief treatment models were more work for staff. With fewer sessions available, goals needed to be established immediately and focused on the client's most pressing problem. Limited sessions also meant more turnover in caseload. For some therapists, brief treatment meant a higher cancel/fail rate and lower productivity. Clients were being seen on less regular schedules, for example, every two weeks or once a month; perhaps they were squeezed in for a first appointment during a prime evening time then scheduled during daytime hours for future appointments. There was less opportunity to develop client relationships of the same depth or duration as in previously used treatment models. The therapist and client worked intensively for several weeks or months on a limited number of issues then ended treatment, with an invitation to the client to return in the future, if need be, for work on other issues.

Organizational Structure

The basic structure of Provident's programs and services remained unchanged with the introduction of managed care services into the agency. Managed PsychCare became an additional program center in the agency's service array. However, at various points along the way, thought was given to creating a subsidiary capitation that would contain the businesslike ventures—the employee assistance, managed care, and customer assistance programs. The 1988 strategic plan went so far as to outline an organizational design with such a corporate subsidiary. However, the effects of having programs that were on the cutting edge of new service developments brought positive and evolutionary changes to the rest of the agency.

Provident manages its client intake through an *information and first appointments department*. All service requests for managed care and traditional counseling services come through a direct line or 800 number for an appointment. The department staff screen for appropriateness, assemble information about the presenting problem, and verify the HMO plan benefits. If outpatient counseling is the appropriate treatment, a first appointment is scheduled at a time and location convenient for the caller. An applicant's request for inpatient or partial hospitalization care is referred for further assessment and authorization to the Managed PsychCare utilization management staff.

Provident's alcohol and drug treatment program, *addiction services*, was restructured as an intensive outpatient treatment program. Its six-week, four-evenings-per-week format provides an alternative to repeated hospitalizations for the chemically dependent person. Clients maintain their normal work routine; family members are integral to the treatment process; the cost is less than that of inpatient care.

An intensive group treatment program for *chronically mentally ill* persons was established. Managed PsychCare found that some of its chronically mentally ill clients were hospitalized for stabilization. Staff believed that regular, consistent contact with a therapist, and the ability to reach a therapist at any time, might prevent the crises that resulted in rehospitalization. The treatment group met three times a week, and the therapists were accessible twenty-four hours a day. During the one year of operation, not a single client in this group required rehospitalization. The program was closed down when too few clients could be identified to operate the group.

Two on-call teams were established. The first team of Managed Psych-Care utilization managers and several Provident therapists provided twenty-four-hour on-call coverage on a rotating basis to hospitals, physicians, and new clients. On-call staff worked on a weekly, rotating basis responding to emergencies from new clients and handling requests for admission or discharge on the weekends or after hours.

A second twenty-four-hour on-call team was established to respond to outpatient client emergencies. Once a client enters treatment with a Provident therapist, after-hours emergencies become the responsibility of the counseling program. The team handles authorization of hospital admissions for overnight, weekends, holidays, and whenever the agency is closed. It is staffed by a weekly, rotating team of Provident therapists who carry pagers and cellular telephones. For example, a client without ready access to his or her therapist might attempt to access a more intense level of care, such as hospital admission when in fact crisis intervention over the telephone and the promise of a Monday appointment could stabilize the client. A client's Friday night or Saturday hospital discharge can also be facilitated by this team.

Staff development has been influenced by the work in managed care. Provident established brief treatment as its priority for staff development. Experts in solution-focused approaches to clinical work have been brought into the agency. Staff have been sent to national seminars on the topic. The chief operating officer (responsible for all of Provident's client services) spent a year providing intensive supervision on brief treatment models to clinical staff in all the counseling centers to help this new approach take hold. Staff development programs now routinely include training in brief therapy models. Solution-focused treatment is included in the curriculum of the agency's training institute. Support staff have also been included in a workshop on managed care so they could enhance their understanding.

Clients Served

In most instances managed care clients were demographically different from persons receiving counseling services paid for by other sources, principally the United Way (see table 3). The gender ratio of identified patients was nearly identical for both groups of clients. There were only one-half as many African Americans represented among the managed care cases as in the United Way–funded counseling clientele. The proportion of African Americans among Provident's traditional counseling clients was above the population percentage for the metropolitan Saint Louis area; the proportion among managed care clients was below the population percentage. This may indicate that African Americans were underrepresented among the employed population that was covered by HMO benefits.

Differences are noted between the age distributions of identified patients. Managed care clients looked remarkably similar to United Way–funded clients. These clients, however, looked markedly younger than clients served through other, non–United Way–funded resources. The geographic residence of clients was very different. Managed care clients were only half as likely to live within the city of Saint Louis. Although they were likely to reside in the county contiguous to the city, managed care clients were increasingly likely to reside in the suburban counties. Therefore, managed care clientele looked remarkable similar to non-managed-care clientele, except for place of residence, which is likely to be suburban rather than within the city.

Performance Criteria and Clinical Outcomes

Provident developed outcome indicators. Several approaches were tested. The first approach focused on customer satisfaction ratings as a mea-

TABLE 3   Demographic Distribution of 1997 Agency Clientele

	Percentage of Clientele			
Characteristic	Total	United Way Funded	Managed PsychCare	Other Non–United Way Funded
Total number served	23,375	3,112	2,292	20,263
Gender				
Female	50%	58%	60%	48%
Male	50%	42%	40%	52%
Race/ethnicity				
African American	54%	26%	15%	61%
Asian	0%	0%	0%	0%
Hispanic	0%	0%	0%	1%
Native American	0%	0%	0%	0%
Caucasian	45%	73%	85%	38%
Other	1%	1%	0%	0%
Age				
< 14	17.9%	22%	21%	14%
15–19	9%	10%	11%	7%
20–34	31%	32%	25%	31%
53–54	37%	32%	36%	40%
55–65	4%	3%	6%	5%
65 >	2%	1%	1%	3%
Annual income				
$0–9,999	59%	49%		64%
$10,000–14,999	16%	17%		15%
$15,000–19,999	8%	11%		7%
$20,000–29,000	7%	10%		5%
$30,000–49,999	4%	3%		4%
$50,000 >	6%	10%		5%
County of Residence				
City of Saint Louis	26%	22%	12%	28%
Franklin	2%	1%	1%	3%
Jefferson	12%	11%	13%	12%
Saint Charles	8%	9%	15%	7%
Saint Louis	38%	41%	48%	37%
Madison	2%	3%	3%	2%
Saint Clair	5%	9%	4%	2%
Other	7%	4%	4%	9%

sure of clinical outcomes. Provident routinely conducted satisfaction surveys of clients served by the agency's programs. During a one-week period each year, survey forms were distributed by secretaries to all counseling clients coming in for services at all locations. Managed PsychCare clients were also contacted through a telephone survey, and results were shared with the HMO.

Several clinical indicators were routinely tracked for managed care cases and reported in the quality improvement process. Failure to meet one or more of the administrative standards would result in loss of revenue to the program. These standards included the following:

Patient and provider access to service as determined by the amount of time or number of rings before the telephone was answered, the rate at which callers abandoned their calls, the average length of time a caller waited on hold, and the immediacy with which a client appointment was scheduled

Utilization rates within a preset range of minimums and maximums

Client satisfaction above a designated minimum level

Relapse and recidivism rates within six months of discharge for adult patients who were rehospitalized

Provident developed quality indicators for each of its programs and services. For counseling and managed care outpatient services, those indicators include the following:

Length of stay (number of sessions) by diagnosis

Degree of goal attainment as determined by the therapist at case closing

In 1997, the results demonstrated that when analyzed by diagnosis, the length of stay for managed care counseling cases was less than for other counseling cases; and in most instances, the degree of goal attainment by diagnosis was *higher* for managed case than for others.

The HMO contract required that a first appointment be scheduled within five working days of the request for service. This meant that Managed PsychCare clients were sometimes the first to be scheduled into scarce and premium appointment times. Managed PsychCare clients waited five to six days on average for their first appointment. Over time, traditional counseling clients' average waiting time for first appointments was reduced from nine working days in 1993 to 5.66 and 5.58 days average wait for counseling and Managed PsychCare clients, respectively, in 1997.

Management and Administration

Several matters dominated the administration of Provident's managed care program: computer services, staff salaries, and accreditation. The increasing need for information to track activity and to manage costs propelled expansion of the agency's management information systems. Managed Psych-Care needed instant access to information about an HMO member's eligibility for service, plan benefits, and prior use of benefits. Staff had to be able to authorize services and track utilization of the authorized treatment. Certain quality indicators necessitated organizational ability to identify cases that fell outside preset parameters. The addition of outcome indicators and claims management drove the refinement of information services for the program.

Agency accreditation was an important element in the selection of Provident to provide services for the HMO. Accreditation by the Joint Commission is seen as an indicator that an organization has met high standards of operation and identified itself with the health care industry. In 1992, Managed Psych-Care was certified as a utilization review agent by the state of Missouri. The cost of accreditations was staggering. However, they were an important aspect of organizational preparation for managed care services.

CONCLUSION

Given the impact that managed care is having on health care, Provident's 1987 board and staff appear to have been prophets. They were opportunistic in their decision to move the agency in the direction of managed care. While they did not know exactly how to do what was initially being asked of them, they sensed the importance that managed behavioral health care would have in the agency's future. They saw an opportunity and the agency's inherent capability to respond.

Several factors contributed to Managed PsychCare's survival and Provident's extended operation in the managed care environment. Managed Psych-Care survived two and a half years longer than was anticipated. This can be attributed to several factors. Some luck is always involved in success stories. Tenacity of the staff was also a major factor. The $2 million operation was good for Provident and very hard to leave. We hung on to the business as long as possible, while not knowing the behavioral health field was moving.

Provident entered the managed care marketplace early. This enabled the organization and the staff to learn while providing the services under contract. We were able to learn and come to understand the technological and interpersonal components of the managed care system while it was in its early stages of construction and development. Understanding the interpersonal components of the system was crucial at various stages in the later years of Managed PsychCare. Building and maintaining interpersonal relationships with key actors and players was vital and cannot be underestimated. As these individuals moved within the purchasers' systems, these relationships were maintained and nurtured. At key points during the mergers, these individuals were able to ensure the continuity of contracting for Provident and Managed PsychCare. This active outreach and interpersonal contact continues to the present.

Early in the contracting arrangements, Provident acquired the technical skills necessary to survive and operate in a competitive business environment. It was beneficial for Provident to learn the new philosophy and methods early in the shift to managed care. In particular, the organization bought technology for operating its financial, quality improvement, and measurement systems. This purchasing of information technology and expertise enabled the organization to operate a high-level, sophisticated monitoring and assurance system. As a result the agency is better prepared in areas like brief treatment and outcome measurement. It is hoped these experiences will better position Provident to survive health care reform in all its forms.

Finally, ongoing monitoring of the marketplace and others' business performance was crucial. This environmental surveillance enabled the organization to adjust to the marketplace and its changes in a timely fashion. Monitoring and scanning were accomplished principally through interpersonal relationships.

The following were among the characteristics Provident Counseling needed in order to take the plunge into managed care:

An entrepreneurial spirit—willingness to take a calculated risk and tolerance for the bumpy ride inherent in any new venture. The board, the executive, and the senior staff needed to share this spirit.

No fear of competition—confidence that agency services can stand up against competitive forces and assurance that managed care services are relevant to the agency's mission. Experience with employee assistance and other competitive contracts were good preparation.

Confidence in the product—services are supervised, staff is trained, the quality of care is closely monitored. The agency has improved, and quality has been enhanced through accreditation. Family service agencies are well prepared in this way.

Provident's experience suggest several recommendations for agencies considering a move into managed behavioral health care:

1. For a family service agency, it is okay *not* to get involved in managed care. Even though a majority of counseling services will be provided in that venue, family agencies have a broader mission and greater capabilities, which offer many other opportunities for community service. There is likely to continue to be a variety of markets for counseling and other services for which a family agency could prepare itself.

2. Obtain brief treatment training for the organization's staff. Identify those staff willing to join the agency in this venture and work with them first. Other staff are likely to come along as the future direction becomes clearer to them.

3. Discover the managed care groups active in your community and seek to become a provider for them. There are any number of possible relation-

ships with HMOs, EAPs, national and regional behavioral health care firms, insurance companies, and the like. Offer to provide their after-hours and weekend coverage; be their on-call or crisis telephone services.

4. Establish program performance indicators that are focused on the results of treatment. What can the behavioral health care company expect to get for its money? What results can be expected?

5. Develop good cost information on programs. Seek to reduce operational and program costs to enhance competitiveness.

6. Experiment with utilization management of agency cases. Develop criteria for service, use a treatment authorization approach, manage the cases to track improvement, use alternative treatment methods.

CHAPTER 7

A Partnership of Community Provider Organizations for Behavioral Health Care

Lloyd H. Sidwell

President and Chief Executive Officer,
Family Resources, Inc., Houston

Texas "culture" is steeped in the boom-bust experiences of the oil industry. In particular, Houston experienced phenomenal growth and speculative entrepreneurialism from the 1960s through the early 1980s, an economic depression in the middle to late 1980s, and the slow beginnings of economy recovery and diversification during the 1990s. The Houston area is the fourth largest metropolitan area in the United States, with an increasingly culturally and ethnically diverse population (Anglo 40.6%, African American 27.5%, Hispanics 27.6%, and Asian 4.1%—1990 U.S. census figures).

Family Service Center (FSC) a nonprofit community service organization serving greater Houston areas individuals and families since 1904, is a medium-sized agency with the mission of strengthening individual functioning and enhancing family relationships. With an annual budget of $4 million and a staff of nearly one hundred, FSC provides solution-oriented individual and family treatment services, chemical dependency treatment services for targeted populations, home care services, and a variety of community-based educational and supportive services for children, parents, and families (including specialized school-based social services and case management services for persons and families affected by HIV/AIDS).

In the 1980s FSC provided employee assistance program (EAP) services. Basic one-to-five visit model services were marketed by FSC to Houston-based small to medium-sized employers. By the late 1980s, the agency had approximately $130,000 annually in Houston area EAP contracts. However, given the staff expense required to support the EAP accounts and routine levels of EAP clinical utilization (5% to 6% for programs moderately promoted by employers), the program cost more to maintain than it produced in revenues.

In 1989, FSC's executive director of twenty-seven years retired, and I was selected from outside the organization as the new chief executive. With my previous experience as the chief executive of a community mental health center in Illinois, and my understanding of the impending changes for the 1990s in behavioral health care systems, a plan soon emerged that focused on establishing the agency's niche as a service provider organization for a variety of payers, including outside EAP/managed care contractors. In addition to being a provider of outpatient treatment services, FSC's strategy for the 1990s included joining with other selected community service organizations to venture in managed behavioral health care on a substate or statewide basis. The remainder of this chapter describes the establishment and operational experiences of such a multiorganizational partnership venture.

DEVELOPMENT OF A MANAGED BEHAVIORAL HEALTH CARE PARTNERSHIP

Historical Context

Prior to my arrival in Houston in 1989, executives from five mental health/mental retardation centers in nonmetropolitan communities throughout east Texas collaborated informally on various projects to improve the mental health/mental retardation service system for their constituents. These centers had annual individual budgets of up to $15 million. As quasi-governmental entities, they receive most of their funding from the Texas Department of Mental Health and Mental Retardation, and their boards of directors are appointed by county government. The centers had worked together to return institutionalized, mentally ill clients to their community and had established joint training programs for their staff. Several of the centers had small EAP programs and had ventured into other entrepreneurial projects. By 1989, the five mental health/mental retardation center executives had preliminary discussions about venturing together as an east Texas consortium to position their centers as managed behavioral health care providers for private-pay community clients.

The center executives recognized that if east Texas was to become the focus for a substate delivery network, it would be necessary to include in the network an organization serving the Houston metropolitan areas. However, the mental health/mental retardation center serving the Houston metropolitan area had not usually joined the other east Texas centers in their collaborations. The size of the Houston area center (an approximately $80 million annual budget) and the complexities of serving the massive urban population led to its focusing exclusively on the poorest and most disturbed of the public population. Resources for, or interest in, entrepreneurial ventures were not on the Houston center's agenda.

Because of common membership in several national mental health organizations and my related ten years of experience as an executive of a community mental health center in Illinois, the five center executives contacted me to discuss further the concept of a managed care venture that would include FSC as the Houston-based partner. Early exploratory discussions revealed our agreement that managed care was the future direction of the financing and structuring of behavior health care delivery. As the group met on several occasions in later 1989 and early 1990, the following judgments regarding the emerging managed care environment and the future viability of our community organization in a changing industry were articulated.

Our Organizations Must Be Players in the Developed Managed Care Business.   Our judgment was that to be uninvolved would mean, in the short-term and long-term, being left out of critical developing systems of both behavioral health care financing and delivery. While we were uncertain of the intricacies that would characterize emerging financing and delivery systems within both commercial markets and the public care arena (Medicaid/Medicare and other publicly funded services), we believed it was better to be involved in change than wait to be affected by changes. Therefore, positioning our organizations to compete in the changing market became our primary rationale for pursuing active participation in managed care.

Our Community Centers Should Be Positioned for Maximum Market Share as Service Providers.   During the 1980s there had been an increase in the conversion of general hospital beds to psychiatric and substance abuse treatment units operated predominantly by proprietary providers. As managed care began restricting reimbursement for inpatient care, and as several national and Texas-based scandals revealed questionable practices with the proliferation of inpatient units, late in the decade proprietary providers began to shift their attention to outpatient program development. Community service agencies began facing new competition for outpatient clients.

With the clear understanding that our organizational missions and primary expertise were as community-based service providers of treatment and supportive services, our individual agency strategies were understandably focused on service delivery. Therefore, we believed it important to engage in ventures that reinforced this role as service provider, especially in light of the increasing competition from proprietary providers.

Management, Marketing, and Sales Operations of EAP/Managed Care Must Be Separate from the Operations of Our Service Provider Organizations.   Those of us involved in the EAP business had heard from corporate customers and competitors that when we both sold EAP service products and provided treatment services, we were perceived as lacking the necessary separation of roles or responsibility appropriate for an "arm's length" or monitoring relationship. The integrity of the arm's length relationship between the business of sales and management of EAP/managed care products, on one side, and the actual delivery of client services, on the other, was perceived to affect the quality of utilization management and the creditability of evaluative measures.

For example, FSC both managed EAP products for Houston area businesses (after having sold them) and provided clinical services for employees and their dependents accessing the EAP benefit. As we began to explore with employers the possibility of expanding the traditional one-to-five visit EAP service into a comprehensive managed care service, some employers expressed a desire for separation of utilization management and service delivery functions to assure utilization consistent with service need. As area employers began to be approached by regional and national EAP/managed care companies, and we began experiencing competition for our existing contracts, we considered how FSC could stay in the business as an active provider organization while separating ourselves from sales and management functions.

Our Traditional Catchment Areas Should Be Extended to Substate, Statewide, and Regional Markets.   Although our community centers were traditionally bound to local service or catchment areas, EAP/managed care systems in the 1990s had to be organized in broader terms. To be competitive in selling EAP/managed care products even to medium-sized companies, it appeared to be critical to participate in an expanded area provider network. Many Houston and Dallas oil, natural gas, and drilling corporations, for instance, had employees outside those metropolitan areas. Company purchasers informed us that access to services was an increasingly critical component to receipt of EAP/managed care contracts. Therefore, we believe it important to broaden our geographic perspective.

We also understood the Texas culture, that is, a prevailing preference for doing business with "inside Texas" companies. We believed a Texas-based EAP/managed care company "owned" by existing Texas organizations would have a competitive advantage. We also thought that because some of our agency board members represented management within major employers, we might be able to extend those relationships to help position our EAP/managed care venture for potential business.

The Integrity and Constituency of Our Community Centers Must Be Protected.   While extending our business venture to a statewide market, we did not want to compromise the established roles and reputations we had in our local communities. This consideration was critical for the mental health/mental retardation centers, which had a defined service constituency of severe and chronic populations. Similarly, while not bound within a catchment area like the mental health/mental retardation centers, FSC had ninety years of Houston area history and reputation critical to private fund-raising and ongoing integrity with the United Way. Establishing a collaborative effort allowed us to participate in a business venture more broadly targeted than our centers' local service focus while preserving the local identity and service markets of our community provider organizations.

We Must Share Resources in Order to Form and Operate a Viable, Competitive Venture.   Initial capitation of a start-up company was beyond the individual financial capacity of any one community organization. However, collectively we could capitalize the venture and lend our separate organizational and service delivery expertise to the venture's success.

We Must Take Risks.   It became apparent early in our planning that the success of a start-up company was not guaranteed. The primary risk for our organizations was the loss of our investment in the partnership. A secondary risk was the possibility of negative publicity with funding sources and the public either because they misunderstood our plans or because they disapproved of our engaging in such an entrepreneurial venture. Additionally, there were personal and professional risks for the executives. While we were not investing our personal funds to capitalize the venture, the center executives were taking individual risks. We risked our credibility with our boards in soliciting their endorsement of the venture, and our venture's failure could compromise each board's confidence in its executive leadership.

Early Development, Middle to Late 1990

We had now reached the point at which expenditures other than our individual meeting time and expense were necessary. Should we proceed with the formal organization of a joint venture, we would have expenses for market consultation and legal representation. To proceed, each of five community centers entered into a contract with the sixth centers, which would serve as the fiscal agent in contracting for initial consultative services for the groups. All six organizations invested $20,000 from their operating reserves, providing pooled resources of $120,000 to initiate planning for our partnership.

With these assessments completed, the center executives believed we needed expert guidance to assess the practicality of our venture. A local management firm was selected to help us develop a request for proposals to be used in soliciting the market guidance of a major health care consulting group. We anticipated that a major health care consulting group would provide us with an analysis of the emerging managed behavioral health care industry and the likelihood of our venture's success. The request for proposals was developed and sent to major consulting firms; we received responses from a half-dozen firms doing business in the east Texas market. We invited the four firms with the most comprehensive initial responses to present to us a summary of market data and their plan for feasibility consultation.

We were surprised to discover that the presentations and plans presented by the selected firms confirmed our original assumptions and assessments and added little to our self-conceived plans. Each of the respondent firms endorsed our concept and offered to "join us" in realizing the goals of our venture. Following the four proposal presentations, the center executives concluded that not only was our concept good but that we knew as much, or more, about the EAP/managed care business as did those now wishing to help us. We decided not to contract with a consulting firm but rather to move forward ourselves to develop a six-organization joint venture.

Organizational Issues

Because of the structures of our community centers, the type of incorporation (either nonprofit or for-profit) and the type of governance structure of the capitation were critical decisions. As a private nonprofit organization, FSC was interested in protecting its long-standing charitable (exempt) status. The five mental health/mental retardation centers, as quasi-public entities with boards appointed by county government and having contractual relationships with the Department of Mental Health and Mental Retardation, were concerned that appropriate separation exist between themselves and the partnership.

One of Houston's preeminent law firms was contracted to advise us on the preferred organizational structure for our venture. With additional advice from the community centers' legal counsel, we determined that each community center should form an affiliated for-profit organizational partnership (see figure 1) under a provision in the Texas law providing for limited liability partnerships. Each community-center-affiliated partner organization would have equal stake in the partnership company by contributing equally to its capitalization. Any future profits would be divided among the partner organizations and distributed to the community centers for support, as locally determined, of their social mission. Governance of the partnership would rest with the partners as represented by the six community center executives, who assumed responsibility as the partnership's board of directors. It was further determined that one of the partner organizations, and its chief executive, would assume responsibility as "managing partner" (a role similar to chairperson of the board). These arrangements would enable the community centers to maintain arm's-length relationships between themselves and the managed care venture, have the flexibility to adding or deleting partners, and minimize liability of our local organizations.

FIGURE 1 Joint Venture Organizational Structure

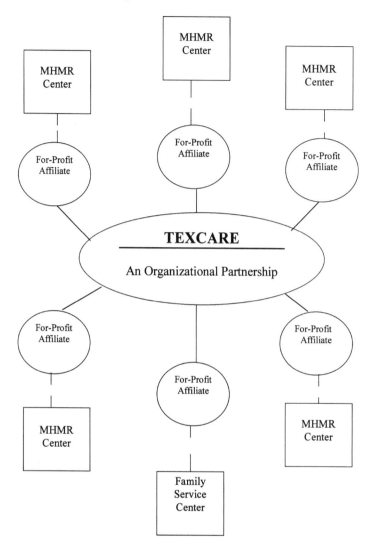

TexCare: From Idea to Incorporation

With an organizational partnership the recommended model, three critical developmental hurdles remained to be passed. First, endorsement by the Department of Mental Health and Mental Retardation was needed in order to provide legitimacy for local mental health/mental retardation center participation. Second, each local community center board of directors needed to formally endorse the venture's concept and then form its affiliated-for-profit entity. Finally, a contribution of funding beyond the original $20,000 was needed from each center as start-up capital for the venture.

The endorsement of the state department was considered a priority, necessarily preceding actions by mental health/mental retardation center boards. Without at least the passive endorsement of the department, the center executives worried that local constituency groups might rush to the inappropriate conclusion that the center's involvement in such a venture was without sanction or diverted public funding from priority programs for severe and chronic populations. A meeting was set with the Texas mental health and mental retardation commissioner to brief him on the proposed venture. Several center board members and members of the commissioner's staff, in addition to the center executives, participated in a several-hour briefing. At the conclusion of the meeting, the commissioner, an experienced professional with a broad view of the challenges facing the mental health/mental retardation centers, endorsed the plans—adding the advice that numerous, mostly critical, eyes would be on us. He encouraged us to proceed with our venture and challenged us to focus our efforts on an enterprise emphasizing quality—the same focus that had already been demonstrated in these centers' operations. Understanding that our venture might well serve as a model for future collaborative and public-private efforts, he told us to "make sure to do it well!"

The center executives continually informed their respective boards of directors about the informal preorganizational efforts regarding the possible joint venture. Each board had previously approved the initial contribution and expenditures for contracting services. With both the specific recommendations of legal counsel regarding organizational structure and the endorsement of the state commissioner, we believed it was time to move forward with each center's formal endorsement of the venture, and for each to create a for-profit affiliate necessary to join the organizational partnership.

Our chosen strategy was to bring together representatives of each center's board for a one-day informational meeting. It was held in a large hotel meeting room at the Dallas–Fort Worth airport (neutral "turf"). The agenda was purposefully structured. Several of the center executives gave presentations on the developing phenomenon of managed care, our developmental efforts, and the venture's significance to the future financial and operational viability of our local centers. Legal counsel attended the meeting and presented the rationale and recommended structure for our joint venture. The agenda left time for both a formal question/response period and informal discussion over lunch. There were many questions, especially about the formation of the for-profit affiliates and the organizational partnership. Legal counsel had consulted with several of the mental health/mental retardation centers' legal counsel prior to the joint meeting. Those counsel were also in attendance to address questions and allay fears. The all-day meeting adjourned with our goals achieved: our local board members were not informed advocates fro the joint venture and were armed with answers to the questions that would understandably accompany discussion by the local boards of directors.

Prior to the centers' board meetings, the executives met to finalize a proposed business plan calling for capital investment by each organization in the partnership. The plan called for a total capital investment of $480,000, which we believed would cover the start-up costs already incurred and the cost of conducting business until earned revenues would cover operational costs. This required an investment of $80,000 from each organization ($60,000 in addition to the original $20,000 contribution for initial start-up expenses). The business plan projected our new company breaking even by the end of the third year and earning a return on our investments beginning in the fourth.

Over several months in late 1990, each center's board approved the formation of its for-profit affiliate organizations and the capital investment for the joint venture. Each center generated the investment funds in its own manner, with most having enough cash reserves generated from private revenues to document the nonexpenditure of public funds for this purpose. (FSC generated its $60,000 share of the capital investment through a loan from its affiliated Family Service Foundation.) Legal counsel filed the necessary partnership documents with the Texas Secretary of State's Office and the respective counties in which the community centers conducted business. We applied for a national "registered mark" for our chosen company name.

With the initial capitalization of the venture, we moved ahead with the selection of an experienced professional to serve as TexCare* chief executive. To advertisements placed in the Houston and Dallas newspapers, we received more than one hundred responses. The center executives interviewed several candidates and selected an individual who had extensive experience with a major managed care company. Our selected executive joined TexCare effective February 1991. Within several months the formal partnership structure was in place and TexCare was ready to begin business.

Development of TexCare, 1991–1992

The partnership executive elected me as the managing partner for the initial phase of our venture's development. During the first year our tasks revolved around organization of the company's internal operations, formation of a provider network, securing of initial business, and beginning delivery of services. As initial managing partner, I worked closely with the chief executive to put in place the internal organizational structure necessary to conduct EAP/managed care business. Forming the legal structure for the company, securing Texas licensures to conduct business as a "third-party administrator" and "utilization review organization," and establishing a reputation required

---

*Not the actual name.

an extensive time commitment from both of us. Public relations and promo-
tional materials were developed, the beginnings of an infrastructure to serve
our contractual clients was established, and contracting sales with small and
medium-sized employers were initiated.

During our first year, TexCare and its chief executive were located in
FSC's administrative office in Houston. This facilitated the coordination of
developmental efforts between the managing partner and the chief executive.
As the growing operation's space needs increased, and with several of our corporate clients headquartered in the Dallas area, TexCare's office site was
moved to the Dallas–Fort Worth metroplex after the first year. The chief executive hired several clinical and additional support staff and formed TexCare's
provider network through Texas and the surrounding states.

TexCare's initial product line consisted of a variety of EAP service
options. They ranged from a minimal one-to-three-visit model to an eight-to-
twelve-visit model. We expanded the business by selling a wider range of services to our primary customers. With a third-party administrator's license we
provided claims adjudication services for an employer's complete mental
health insurance claims. We increasingly offered our corporate customers utilization management services to control their employees' access to, or prolonged stays in, inpatient psychiatric care. We tracked the resulting savings
that our utilization management services produced in the employer's mental
health insurance costs and used this information when working with the
employer on the annual renewal and expansion of the EAP/managed care benefit.

The provider network was developed to assure response capability in
those communities and areas where we were selling our service products. Several of our initial corporate customers were oil and gas companies with
employees in multiple locations, so it was necessary for TexCare to have a
provider network covering most of Texas and targeted areas in the bordering
states. Our provider network consisted of both individual providers (private
practice psychiatrists, psychologists, and masters-degree/licensed therapists)
and institutional providers (agencies, large practice groups, hospitals, and
other service facilities). Our community service organizations were considered preferred providers, but not the only providers, for the outpatient services we provided in our communities. Our centers and clinicians had to meet
the same criteria as other approved providers and were used by TexCare only
if we were continually able to provide services that were accessible and satisfying to consumers.

Our business plan indicated that expenses would exceed earned revenues for the several years of start-up, until such time as our contract business
base was large enough to fully support operational costs. In the competitive
EAP/managed care market, the growth of our contractual business developed
more slowly then originally projected. Although our revenue from sales during the fist two years was below projections, we were able to keep expenses

below initial projections and thus maintain a portion of the initial capital investment to sustain operations into the third year. Slow but steady growth in sales and close fiscal management allowed TexCare to conclude its first two years of business having expended only approximately $380,000 of our $480,000 original capital investment. We ended 1992 with a growing book of business amounting to approximately $500,000 in annual contractual sales, a spreading reputation for quality service, and $100,000 in operating revenues.

Operational Changes in TexCare and Its Environment, 1993

At the beginning of TexCare's third year of operation, the partners met to take stock of the venture. Our goal was to evaluate the impact of a changing behavioral health care market. We had a sense that the market had changed significantly during the intervening years, and that we needed to adjust our strategies if the company was to continue to grow.

While the market dynamics that existed in early 1993 appeared to be identical to those that existed when we conceived our venture in 1990, continuing and rapid change in the health care industry was an increasingly important political and business reality. A newly elected national administration had assumed office, increasing health care costs continued to threaten governmental and business economics, and health care reform was on the agenda both of public and of private business. The health care industry was undergoing restructuring and consolidation. EAP/managed care companies were being caught in the beginning frenzy of rapid and sweeping change. As a small start-up company, TexCare was increasingly competing with other regional managed care companies that began to target the behavioral health care market. The large and relatively undeveloped managed care market of Texas was beginning to receive the attention of major insurance and managed care companies that had not previously viewed Texas as a place to target. The financial resources the major companies brought to the market were ominous to a small company like TexCare.

We believed there was both threat and continuing opportunity in this changing environment. We observed that TexCare was a new and small player in a business increasingly controlled by large, consolidated managed care corporations—Medco Behavioral Care, United States Behavioral Health, Green Spring Mental Health, and the like—and their competitive business practices. From TexCare's experience in the marketplace, we knew that the price of managed behavioral health care products was being driven down by competition. Capitated rates for traditional EAP products were steadily decreasing. Consequently, margins were lower (traditional one-to-three-visit EAP product rates declined from over $2.00 per employee per month to under $1.40 within this time period). With price competition increasingly governing the selection of behavioral health care contractors, it was apparent that control of costs was necessary to ensure viability in the changing market. Managed care companies, such as TexCare and its larger, richer, more sophisticated regional and national competitors, had to control operational costs to remain competitive and attractive to the private businesses that continued to be the primary purchasers of health care benefits and services. We were uncertain whether TexCare could compete effectively over time; however, we wanted to continue collecting information to help us make tat ultimate determination.

While our early entry into the field in Texas was a benefit, the partner executives believed that we needed to increase the book of business so that the costs of competitive operation could be spread. Increased attention to both sales and internal operations would be necessary if we were to accomplish this growth. One of our partner executives had moved to the Dallas area and was available to provide enhanced partners oversight. This partner executive also had a "business" rather than a human services background. Therefore, we changed the managing partner assignment to the Dallas-based colleague. By changing managing partners, we initiated a dual strategic agenda of controlling the operating costs of the company (which we believed were not adequately within management's control) and expanding contract sales (which we believed had not risen to the challenge of our competitors).

Our refocusing worked well. During 1993, the partner executives gained needed insight into the strengths and weaknesses of TexCare's management and operations. Our primary strength was that corporate customers were satisfied with our performance. These customers renewed contracts with us and, in some cases, extended their business. Our provider network (over three hundred individual and organizational providers) was being maintained and was well managed. To control costs we initiated limits on provider billing that improved our accounts payable management. Profitability was difficult because of the overall inefficiencies of our internal operations. However, we became increasingly aware of the inadequacy of our management information system. We conducted our service business and processed our financial claims and payments with minimal computerization. While we hoped that increased sales would provide improved economies of scale, sales were not increasing at a pace that allowed us to achieve these projections.

In 1993, we reached the breakeven point by both enhancing sales and controlling operating costs. With annual contract revenues approaching $600,000, we were nearing our goal of operating within earned revenue. Once again, we were in accord with the target of our original business plan. We were relatively optimistic that our company could produce a small operating profit in its fourth year.

Reassessing the Future

In early 1994, with guarded optimism about our future, the partner executives met for a planning retreat to once again review our venture and the

EAP/managed care business environment. Forcing ourselves to look beyond current operations and our collective desire to succeed with the joint venture, we questioned TexCare's future profitability. Three specific dynamics raised doubts about the long-term viability to the company.

The Market Environment Had Changed More, and More Rapidly, Than We Had Anticipated, Because of Pending Health Care Reform and Health Sector Consolidation.   In less than four years, the rapid growth of managed care had reshaped health care financing and delivery systems. Consolidation of managed care entities had begun. Texas had become a target for development and investment by the major managed care players in the industry. We believed it would become more and more difficult for small EAP/managed care companies to compete in a business environment increasingly dominated by large managed care companies (whether insurance companies themselves or health maintenance organizations entering the behavioral health care business).

Price Competition Was Increasing within the Managed Behavioral Health Care Market.   Guidelines for pricing that had previously been the basis for bidding on EAP/managed care contracts were no longer valid. Contract reimbursement rates were dropping. The company had to further control its costs to compete effectively as a vendor in the more price-competitive environment. Operating costs had to be further reduced to produce even minimal profit margins.

Payers were demanding more account services (claims adjudication and payment, utilization management services, detailed account reporting, and so forth). Managed care companies required management information systems that were effective in producing data to meet payer demands. Greater sophistication in management information systems would require a substantial increase in capital investment.

Product Competition Was Increasing within the Managed Behavioral Health Care Market.   Purchasers of EAP/managed care products were demanding a broader, deeper product array. Purchasers were demanding provision of "on-time" response and service access. They were also beginning to demand a full continuum of care that addressed consumer needs and that would integrate with physical health care. Finally, purchasers were also demanding that the continuum of care include an increasingly sophisticated array of client service options to assure, whenever appropriate, out-of-hospital care.

These dynamics led us to question continued viability of a small, undercapitalized managed care company like TexCare. To compete in an environment increasingly controlled by major, consolidated companies would be difficult without a significant expansion in our infrastructure. The marketing and sales force would have to be expanded, the capacity of information systems would have to be enhanced, and service delivery processes would have to be expanded greatly while becoming more evident.

We concluded that we had two options. We could merge, venture, or ally with another managed behavioral health care enterprise, thereby adding to our size and strength as a competitor for contractual business with developing Texas health plans. Or we could sell the business to a major health plan or integrated managed care company, thereby strengthening and adding value to that health plan or managed care company's Texas and Southwest operations. In both scenarios, we would seek to preserve the preferred provider status of our local community service organizations and to optimize the return on our original financial investment.

Few individuals or entities were interested in investing our existing operation. However, because of the fervor of merger and acquisition activity in the industry, TexCare had a plethora of suitors. We had $650,000 in annual contracts, which was a respectable book of business. We had developed a provider network throughout the Southwest. We had a core staff experienced in managing behavioral health care. These were valuable assets for a company wishing to either enter or expand in the Texas market. Several managed care companies expressed interest, and a few made proposals for either merger or acquisition.

In the middle of 1994, we received an acquisition offer that we believed was worth our serious consideration. The offer met our two requirements. A major managed care company offered to acquire TexCare's assets and continue the partner organizations as preferred providers in its Texas contracted provider network. The acquisition would take the partners out of the sales and account services business but would keep the community agencies in the provider business. An additional benefit was that the offer would leave the organizational partnership as a "shell" company to be developed as we might wish in the future.

We entered a due diligence process with the potential purchaser that extended over seven months. The real market value of TexCare was determined. Following negotiations over contractual interests, staff interests, and final purchase price, our five years as a start-up managed behavioral health care enterprise ended on February 28, 1995, with the sale of TexCare's assets and name. After legal and insurance expenses associated with the sale and conclusion of our business, the net sale revenue returned the majority of each partner organization's original financial investment. The partner executives again met in May 1995 to assess retrospectively our experiences as an organizational partnership in behavioral health care. The essence of our assessment follows.

ANALYSIS OF THE EXPERIENCE

The experience of owning and directing a private managed care enterprise has been invaluable. This learning laboratory provided operational insight for our community service organizations into the realities of collaboration. It taught us lessons in strategic business management. It kept us aware of the rapid and substantial changes occurring in the behavioral health care and human service industry. It sharpened and strengthened our executive abilities.

In my judgment, being an observer is an inadequate substitute for being a player in this rapidly changing business. During my attendance at a national behavioral health care conference, I heard a litany of unsolicited anecdotes from attendees expressing either their false sense of comprehension of the upheaval in our industry or their bewilderment at our industry's nebulous future. The TexCare experience provided us with neither false security nor relief from anxiety about the future of behavioral health services or our community service organizations' viability in a changed service system. TexCare did, however, give us the opportunity to be part of the structural and delivery transitions under way in health care in general, and behavioral health care in particular.

The Collaborative Experience

Contemporary human service industries have adopted collaboration as the 1990s approach to efficient provision of services. Most private and public requests for proposals promote collaboration as a necessary component in any proposed service delivery model. However, few organizations or their executives have operational understanding of, or experience with, the intricacies of managing and operating a service venture through a model of interorganizational and interpersonal cooperation. The traditional model for most human service and health care organizations has been to build a single organization in size and influence. Community service colleagues have been, at least privately, competitors for funding resources. Even when thrust into arrangements where collaboration is expected, many executives and their colleagues tend to operate in parallel rather than integrating for collective strength.

Our shared leadership in TexCare taught us lessons in executive cooperation and collaboration. We did well in most regards but fell short in assuming some of the joint responsibilities. On the positive side, the planning of our joint venture was an excellent example of interorganizational collaboration. Together the agency executives articulated and agreed on the salient issues, the planning process, and initial implementation strategies. We used the diversity of our service delivery and executive experiences to speed the development of an implementation plan for our new venture. Our shared perceptions of the environment and vision for action enabled us to take advantage of what we all sensed to be a closing window of opportunity in the early 1990s to develop a regional EAP/managed behavioral health care company. We were one of the first collaborations of community service providers to actively enter the managed care business.

The partner executives met often to deal with a developmental agenda that required both deliberation and executive judgment. The early enthusiasm of the creative experience provided the essential energy for an atmosphere of excitement about our venture. TexCare's hired executive shared this initial excitement and enthusiasm. We moved ahead quickly with the operationalization of our vision of a Texas-owned, Texas-managed behavioral health care enterprise.

Unfortunately, the initial enthusiasm and energy invested in the venture could not be sustained. As the joint venture matured, we had increasing difficulty working together toward the achievement of common goals. While the working relationships never became adversarial, over time we simply worked less effectively as a team. The initial phases of developing our enterprise were witness to a productive team experience. The continuing implementation of such an entrepreneurial venture required additional, adaptive characteristics of collaboration that were more difficult to produce. As we implemented the structure and operation of TexCare, our work changed from creative endeavor to operational responsibility for managing a company and staff from a distance. Some of the partner executives progressively lost direct contact with, and involvement in, our joint venture. The managing partner was increasingly the focal point of both delegated responsibility and scapegoating for persistent operational difficulties. In my judgment, our collaborative cohesiveness dissolved, and we became less effective in providing leadership for the company.

Concurrent with our collective oversight of TexCare, the partner executives were individually confronting the early 1990s challenges to their community service organizations' survival. Decreases in a variety of public funding, increasing individual and social service needs, together with growing chaos and unpredictability of health care reform, regularly diverted our individual time and energy from TexCare to more immediate, local agency issues. The partner executive began to delegate operational control to executive management without the tight, directional oversight and monitoring necessary to track a start-up's progress. We were increasingly willing to let executive management develop the company. This proved to be a major shortcoming in our execution of our ownership role and governance responsibility.

Lessons of Business Management

The quality of executive management now required for a nonprofit organization is well documented in the literature. No longer can the successful nonprofit executive have skills restricted to charitable vision and mission. The nonprofit executive must be able to manage and balance the organization's mission and constituencies, on the one hand, and its business operation, on the other. The TexCare experience provided us with hard-learned lessons in business management from the perspective of a leading stakeholder in a for-profit enterprise.

The partner executive's careers were located in nonprofit, community service organizations. After years of leadership in our provider organizations, we found ourselves on the other side of the table as directors of a for-profit enterprise. As the TexCare board, we learned to view provider organizations as market commodities because our company was purchasing services in an environment teeming with nonprofit and proprietary providers. As a purchaser, we observed and welcomed the developing competition among these provider organizations. This opposite view helped us understand the strengths and weaknesses of our own provider organizations relative to the trends, issues, and changing demands of purchasers and the provider market.

We learned quickly that margins and profits guide judgments in the competitive business environment. As outside directors, our view was not that of management—our view in our home community agencies—but that of shareholders exercising the responsibilities of ownership. While TexCare's management staff emphasized relative issues of high-quality care (customer satisfaction, utilization review, and so forth), our governance roles and responsibilities became focused on the financial viability and competitiveness of our company.

Personally, I found this experience directly applicable to the changing demands of executives leadership in my community service organization. I was better able than before to focus FSC's management attention on necessary management strategies for today's nonprofit providers, that is, on business issues of productivity and earned revenues. This concentration of energy and attention has yielded greater management efficiency. FSC's internal structure was streamlined to permit a more rapid response to changing demands. We eliminated several programs that were financial burdens on our organization because reimbursement rates were inadequate to cover both the costs of providing services and the additional prescriptions of government bureaucracy. We may have foreseen the necessity of these changes. However, I believe the TexCare experience helped me and my colleagues make judgments by knowing how our competitors in the proprietary environment think and act.

The business management lessons learned from sitting on the board of a private venture have helped prepare our agency for the substantial changes in public and private funding of behavioral health care and social services. When our local agency was confronted with a significant reduction in United Way and service fee revenues in the early 1990s, we were able to address the change process from a business management perspective rather than relying on traditional nonprofit methods. Agency management and board addressed the threat by focusing on financial solvency when confronting the many issues of organizational downsizing. The parallels between the business realities confronting TexCare and those at FSC were too obvious to ignore. Good business practices make sense in both for-profit and nonprofit organizations, and in both they are a necessity.

In addition to learning to exercise financial judgment, we were exposed to other aspects of business different from our experiences in nonprofit organizations. In our roles as TexCare partners, our experiences and relationships were increasingly with leaders from health care and other businesses. We came to view issues of human resource allocation and management, customer relations, management information systems, and organizational affiliation or acquisition from a different perspective than our predominantly nonprofit, human service orientation. Our new relationships, and perspectives, presented a learning challenge appropriate in both a changing industry and changing times.

CONCLUSION

For FSC and me, the partnership of community provider organizations for managed behavioral health care was worth both the human and financial resources invested. This conclusion is generally shared by my center executive colleagues. My increased understanding of operations and future trends in managed care strengthened FSC as a community service provider. My direct experience in managing a for-profit venture enhanced my executive leadership abilities. And FSC realized a reasonable return on its financial investment.

The changes occurring in the behavioral health care industry are staggering. We have already witnessed rapid change in the entire delivery system and in methods of practice, especially the phenomenal decrease in inpatient utilization. Further changes are inevitable. Provider organizations are consolidating, and these consolidations will continue as the industry confronts excess capacity in outpatient services. Controlled practice protocols with care management focused on documentable outcome from minimal intervention are increasingly driving treatment.

It is my judgment that FSC is now better prepared to provide behavioral health care services than many similar organizations. Our five-year venture with TexCare gave me and my center executive colleagues experience that will enable us to continually confront, and adjust to, the changing environment. This learning will continue to benefit our community service organizations.

CHAPTER 8

The Continuum of Care in Children's Behavorial Health Care

Robert Barker

Executive Director,
Southwest Behavioral Health Systems, Houston

Stephen P. Wernet

Professor, School of Social Service,
Saint Louis University

Almost two decades ago, DePelchin Children's Center, a private, nonsectarian child welfare organization, began a process of organizational change that would result in the eventual development of an integrated and comprehensive continuum of care. In the later stages of that development, managed care principles played a significant role as instruments of service integration.

In the late 1970s and early 1980s DePelchin Children's Center began to study the feasibility of implementing a continuum of care that integrated child welfare and children's mental health services within the organization. We concluded that it was important to develop the continuum in partnership with major, public, child-serving organizations and to prepare for private insurance, managed care opportunities. DePelchin had a long history of providing services through a variety of contracts with public mental health and public child welfare agencies in Houston. Because of DePelchin's programmatic and fiscal size, the organization's decisions, if not agreed to in principle by the public agencies, could have jeopardized its funding. In addition, the way DePelchin decided to deliver services, again because of its size, would affect overall delivery systems for children's services in Harris County. Leading psychiatrists, social workers, and psychologists were consulted in the design of the continuum, and some general principles were set forth.

In the early 1980s very few agencies in the United States provided both child welfare and children's mental health services. We had a dream that DePelchin Children's Center could be one of the first children's agencies in the United States to develop a combined child welfare and mental health continuum that would truly consider the needs of both the child and the family. The dream sprang from decisions the DePelchin board and management had already made to convert some of the residential program to a residential treatment center for emotionally disturbed children. We believed that the agency's strong tradition as a high-quality child welfare provider would be the base on which mental health services could be developed and integrated with child welfare services. We knew that this would be a major departure from the current models of services that defined children as either in need of child welfare services or in need of children's mental health services.

FRAGMENTATION IN CHILDREN'S SERVICES

The evolution of child welfare services in the United States has been both incremental and disjointed. Orphanages were the first type of care used for orphaned, abandoned, and abused children. They were followed by the development of adoption and foster care services. Many of the early advocates of adoption and foster care called for an end to orphanages and large, long-term institutions for children. Consequently, well into the 1980s many leaders in the child welfare field felt a need to defend the role of institutions as the best method of care for abused and neglected children.

However, by the 1980s it also became clear that children were being lost in the system and, too often, family reunification was a vain hope. Long-term care, a focus of most child welfare institutions, was targeted for criticism by numerous advocacy groups. The Adoption Assistance and Child Welfare Act of 1980 (PL96–272) and the Family Preservation Act of 1992 were the culmination of major efforts by advocacy groups to end out-of-home care drift. These laws had the goal of ensuring permanent families for children by either returning children to their families of origin, freeing them for adoption, or deterring out-of-home placement by strengthening families of origin. Residential child care providers who did not operate adoption and foster care services were placed in a precarious position.

Unfortunately, divisions developed within the child welfare community itself. These divisions pitted out-of-home care providers, specifically campus-based long-term institutional care providers and foster family care and adoption providers, against residential treatment providers. Amid the disagreements among child welfare professionals, the Child Welfare League of America (CWLA) was unable to provide a unifying voice. Believing that CWLA was neglecting these services (especially for white children), advocates of adoption services established the National Committee for Adoptions. Similarly, believing that CWLA was overcommitted to permanency planning and foster care family services, advocates for long-term child care institutions established the National Association of Homes for Children. Many child welfare and mental health professionals began looking to other disciplines for examples of service models that would reduce the fragmentation and lack of coordination in children's services. The continuum-of-care model, more typical in medicine, was thought to be applicable the identified problems in child welfare and children's mental health.

Lack of coherence and fragmentation also characterized children's mental health services. The community health movement advocated development of community-based mental health centers. The core principle of this movement was that children should be able to receive mental health services on an outpatient basis within the context of their families and communities. Organizations separate from community mental health centers began developing residential treatment centers for emotionally disturbed youth. While the conflict between these two clusters of advocates was less pronounced than in the child welfare field, effective linkage and referral systems were not developed. In summary, professional infighting and competing treatment philosophies contributed to fragmented and incoherent services for children and their families, even though treatment and system design philosophies existed to address both of these issues.

THE CONTINUUM-OF-CARE MODEL

A continuum of care can be defined as an array or uninterrupted and orderly sequence of services for supporting and enhancing the functioning of children and their families. It refers to both a philosophy and an operationalization of services. Philosophically, a continuum of care refers to a clinical environment in which children and their families can easily access any service within the array. When a child and his or her family move among services in a continuum, the move should be relatively easy and there should be continuity of relationship with service providers during the move. This is especially important for children who have experienced prior losses of relationships with family members due to abuse and neglect.

Operationally, a continuum of care requires development of clinical standards or protocols. An organization must develop and use specific criteria that guides staff decision making about the clinical needs of a child and his or her family. A continuum of care must have 1) a full and creative array of services, 2) quick and effective diagnostic and treatment processes, 3) highly individualized treatment planning, 4) an emphasis on least restrictive services, and 5) delivery of care that is oriented toward high-quality outcomes.

Defining the Ideal Continuum of Care

To respond to the care and treatment needs of youth in every community, a comprehensive continuum of care should be designed to prevent child abuse, neglect, and mental health problems to the extent that current technologies are available to do so. In addition, all services generally recognized by professionals in the field as necessary, from least restrictive to most restrictive, should be available in the continuum. Therefore, the following services should be included in a comprehensive continuum:

1. Prevention services that target at-risk families and children

2. Accessible information and referral services

3. Twenty-four-hour crisis intervention services designed to quickly help families deescalate the crisis and engage in the lest restrictive treatment possible

4. Outpatient mental health services

5. Home-based services that use technologies developed in the family prevention and home health care fields

6. Day treatment combined with school-based services

7. Emergency shelter or assessment center

8. Community-based family-style group homes

9. Residential treatment centers

10. Psychiatric hospitals

Organizational and Operational Issues for the Ideal Continuum Care

A continuum of care can be designed and implemented either within one organization or across numerous organizations. A continuum developed by one organization presents many advantages. The organization has complete authority to expand or contract different services within the continuum and can more easily shift financial profits and losses from one service to another. Continua that involve more than one organization, however, may be able to add competence because of the unique programming of several organizations. When an individual organization develops a continuum of care, it is usually for a specific population of children and families defined by either geographic locale or client needs. When an individual organization chooses to develop and implement a comprehensive continuum of care, it must provide most or all of the services described above and apply the same design principles.

A multiorganizational or community continuum of care should be organized in such a way that referral systems and case management systems are designed to make it easy for children and their families to access all appropriate services. Several community models have been developed in recent years. These community models have been designed to improve service accessibility and coordination among providers. They are also designed to control and contain costs and to use the least restrictive services consistent with a client's clinical needs.

INCUBATING THE CONTINUUM-OF-CARE MODEL

Our analysis of child welfare and other systems in the greater Houston metropolitan area led DePelchin Children's Center to design a specific set of services that would constitute a continuum of care for children either in their own home or in out-of-home placement. We believed the continuum of care must be prepared to respond quickly and flexibly to children and families in crisis, adapting whatever services were available to what families or public agencies could afford and were willing to purchase. A basic operational principle of continuum in children's services, and in managed care delivery systems, is a service delivery system that provides the most appropriate service as soon as possible after the need has been identified and to provide no more, and no fewer, services than are needed. Furthermore, we believed that there were clear advantages in combining child welfare services with children's mental health services. Children needing child welfare services have usually been abused, neglected, or abandoned. Frequently, this population of children also has mental health needs requiring treatment. Conversely, many emotionally disturbed children who are not victims of abuse or neglect need services that have been developed primarily within the child welfare field. Consequently, after a literature review and consultation with CWLA, we specified the following services within the continuum of care for children requiring out-of-home placement.

1. A psychiatric hospital for acute, extreme disturbance, when intensive treatment in a secure setting is required
2. A residential treatment center for longer term, less costly, institutional care for the time when the crisis has been ameliorated but the child is too disturbed to live in a community-based group home or in a foster home
3. Therapeutic or regular foster and group homes offering alternative, home-like community living for children whose parents are still too disturbed or disorganized to aid them in their further progress, or for children whose parents will never be able to care for them and for whom adoption is not an option

The for-profit mental health delivery system in Houston in the early 1980s overemphasized the role of psychiatric hospitalization, especially for teenagers. The private child welfare system, with the exception of DePelchin and Houston Achievement Place (a provider of community-based group home care), almost entirely used institutional care as the treatment of choice for abused and neglected children removed from their homes. Therefore, we concluded that the greater metropolitan Houston children's continuum of care would include services that enabled children, whenever possible, to remain with their families or to receive families through adoption. Consequently, we specified the following services for this population:

1. Adoption and postadoption services for infants, older children, and sibling groups

2. Home-based family preservation services in which caseworkers provide intense family-focused services in an effort to prevent unnecessary out-of-home placement

3. Day treatment services for children who can live with their own families or in foster care but who have treatment needs too intense to serve on an outpatient basis

4. Outpatient services to support the child in his adjustment to live in his home, school, and community

The development of an effective child welfare and children's mental health continuum of care within DePelchin would have to occur in the context of the history and the traditions of the organization. The case study that follows describes the context in which the continuum was developed and the steps taken to develop the continuum.

DEPELCHIN CHILDREN'S CENTER: A CASE STUDY

Historical Background

DePelchin Children's Center was founded in Houston, Texas, in 1892 by a nurse, Kezia DePelchin, to care for children orphaned as a result of a yellow fever epidemic. During the 1920s, the agency offered foster care and adoption services as alternatives to institutional care for infants and toddlers. Until 1978 DePelchin provided a range of services including institutional care for dependent and neglected children, foster care, teen pregnancy services, and adoption services.

Minutes from board of directors meeting in the 1920s and 1930s indicate that the organization had a commitment to quality and providing services within the context of national standards. For example, in 1933, the executive director of CWLA provided consultation to DePelchin for the design of new residential cottages. Built in the late 1930s, the cottages were intended to serve smaller groups of children than was typical at that time. Because of their features, some of these buildings were converted to residential treatment units in 1978.

DePelchin began assuming a leadership role in human services in Houston and Texas in the pre–World War II era. It was a founding member of the Houston United Way and supported the development of a state agency for child protective services. Masters-degreed social workers were recruited form out-of-state universities to provide staff professional leadership.

In the 1930s, the DePelchin board of directors recognized the need of African American children for child welfare services. The public child welfare system was seriously underfunded, and most child welfare services were provided by private agencies that served only white children. Funding and recruitment of trained social workers were major obstacles to developing child welfare services in African American communities. In 1938, DePelchin, in partnership with the United Way and a volunteer organization in one of the African American wards of Houston, founded the Negro Child Care Center. This center operated as a separate, segregated division of DePelchin. It served thousands of African American children and their families until the late 1960s when, following the Civil Rights Act, all DePelchin services were racially integrated. Today, largely as a result of these bold steps to serve African American children in the 1930s, DePelchin continues to serve a significant number of children of color.

Throughout the post–World War II period and into the later 1970s, DePelchin continued to be the leading private child welfare agency in Houston and its surrounding communities. The services provided during this era continued to be built around long-term institutional care, foster family care, and adoption services primarily for infants.

Impetus for Change

Although DePelchin continued to be the leading children's agency in Houston during the 1960s and 1970s, the organization failed to keep pace with some of the major changes occurring in private child welfare organizations in the United States. DePelchin's board of directors was reluctant to convert some or all of the agency's basic child care institutional program into a residential treatment program, even though there were no residential treatment programs for children and adolescents in Houston. A 1976 CWLA study of the agency concluded that DePelchin was operating an outdated institutional program serving troubled children and adolescents without adequate clinical services. Senior staff of the Houston United Way read the report and informed the DePelchin board that major changes would have to be made or the United Way would reduce its allocations to the agency. In 1976 the annual United Way allocation for the agency's residential program was $450,000.

The pressure for DePelchin to change increased when a local advocacy organization, CAN-DO-IT (an organization of mental health professionals, influential citizens, and parents of emotionally disturbed children), proposed a joint venture with DePelchin. The joint venture offer included an initial $250,000 to be provided by CAN-DO-IT and subsequent annual gifts to enable DePelchin to operate a residential treatment program for emotionally disturbed children. In 1977 DePelchin and CAN-DO-IT entered into an agreement that resulted in a twenty-two-bed residential treatment center for children. The agreement between the organizations provided that 1) there would be a joint oversight committee to advise the DePelchin board and management about the development and operation of the residential treatment program and 2) three members of the CAN-DO-IT organization would join the

DePelchin board. The joint venture program was opened on the DePelchin campus in 1978.

The joint oversight committee for the residential treatment program consisted of the three new DePelchin board members appointed from the CAN-DO-IT organization, three additional individuals on the CAN-DO-IT board, and three long-standing DePelchin board members. The oversight committee began advocating for significant changes within DePelchin, for services for emotionally disturbed children, and for a role in selecting an outsider to direct the residential treatment program.

The three CAN-DO-IT representatives on the DePelchin Board played major roles in future agency developments. One of the representatives came from an influential family that controlled one of the major Houston newspapers and the largest philanthropic foundation in Houston. Another representative was director of social services for the county hospital district. The third representative was a leading Houston rabbi who chaired the board search committee for a new executive director in 1979.

Resignation of the Executive Director

Although a number of factors were probably involved, the new organizational direction—that is, developing mental health services in tandem with child welfare services—appeared to have played a major role in the decision of the executive director to resign. Two of the seven members of the board executive search committee, including the committee chairperson, had joined the board as CAN-DO-IT representatives. The board clearly expected that DePelchin would become a children's mental health organization as well as a child welfare organization. The first author of this case study began his tenure as executive director in November 1979.

The Strategic Plan

A strategic planning process began during the first quarter of 1980. This board/staff process identified four important issues:

1. Expand the endowment fund to provide earned income that could enable DePelchin to provide mental health and child welfare services for indigent populations.
2. Add a stronger psychiatric component to services.
3. Convert the campus to residential treatment over a three-year period.
4. Develop "step down" services for children in residential treatment such as day treatment and outpatient services, and add these services to the existing array of services when funding becomes available. The decision to add step-down services was in effect a forerunner to the development of a continuum-of-care delivery model.

Implementing the Strategic Plan

Step 1: Endowment Expansion. A $10 million endowment campaign was announced in 1981. Over four years, $8 million of the $10 million goal was raised. The first award was a $5 million foundation grant for mental health services. Soon thereafter, a $1 million endowment award was granted by another foundation to help underwrite the costs of psychiatric residency training at DePelchin. The foundation that awarded the $5 million grant required DePelchin to become accredited by the Joint Commission on the Accreditation of Healthcare Organizations, to employ a psychiatrist to direct the organization's mental health services, and to provide outpatient services to children following their discharge from residential treatment.

DePelchin's board and management believed that the foundation's stipulations were reasonable given the community need for mental health services and the size of the grant. Consequently, the award with its stipulations were accepted by the DePelchin board.

Step 2: A Stronger Psychiatric Component. The decision to develop a medically directed mental health service was unique among private child welfare and mental health organizations in the early 1980s. Several factors led to this decision. First was the foundation's stipulation attached to the $5 million grant. Second was the influence of the two Houston medical schools and their strong public advocacy that DePelchin's mental health services be medically directed. Third was the medical schools' accompanying desire to create training opportunities for psychiatric residents. Fourth was the acute shortage of mental health services for children and adolescents in Houston. (Texas ranked forty-eighth in per capita expenditures of public funds for children's mental health services in 1980.) Consequently, with a $5 million endowment, DePelchin was expected to design the most modern and expert mental health system possible. It was presumed that whatever mental health services were developed by DePelchin would be of high quality. Most DePelchin board members believed that the best way to accomplish this goal would be to have a leading child psychiatrist direct the developing mental health services.

A search committee that included the executive director, DePelchin's board chair, the head of psychiatry at one of the medical schools, and a noted child psychiatrist in the community led the effort to select and employ a Harvard University–trained child psychiatrist with specific training in residential treatment and hospital services. The individual selected had strong interests in developing both a mental health service delivery system for seriously disturbed youth and a strong psychiatric residency training program. In 1985 DePelchin became a training site for Baylor University psychiatric residents.

Step 3: Campus Conversion. During the first two operating years of the new residential treatment program, it became apparent that DePelchin was being asked to treat children who were more emotionally disturbed than origi-nally anticipated. Because there were no other residential treatment options and there were no psychiatric hospital beds for children under 13 in the com-munity, DePelchin frequently admitted children into residential treatment who should have received at least some brief period of stabilization in a psychiatric hospital. Consequently, in 1981, a nine-bed psychiatric hospital for children under 13 was opened on the DePelchin campus. By 1983 the entire campus with the exception of a sixteen-bed emergency shelter facility was converted to residential treatment. The new configuration of the DePelchin Children's Cen-ter consisted of fifty-five residential treatment beds, nine psychiatric hospital beds, and sixteen shelter beds for abused and neglected children.

In the 1980s most children in the psychiatric hospital and the residen-tial treatment program were public agency referrals. In fall 1981 the first con-tract for psychiatric hospital services was signed with an insurance company, Blue Cross. Additional insurance contracts were signed during 1982 and 1983. Some of the insurance companies began purchasing residential treat-ment as step-down services for children following their brief stays in the hos-pital unit. These early endeavors with insurance companies enabled DePelchin to gain experience serving insured populations, which would be helpful to the organization when it entered into care contracts in 1987. Staff learned that unlike the more compliant public sector staff and clients, insured clients were more vocal and more demanding and expected higher quality cus-tomer service from organizations such as DePelchin. Insured clients often complained if they disagreed with treatment protocols. Parents of children were often required by their insurance companies to make copayments and often expected, and even demanded, services that fit their schedules, for example, counseling sessions on evenings and weekends.

Step 4: Developing Step-Down Services. Between 1982 and 1987 there was a continuous push to develop a comprehensive child welfare and children's mental health continuum of care. The process was gradual because of insufficient public funding for these services. Competition from for-profit psychiatric hospitals that also offered residential treatment, day treatment, and outpatient services to insured clients limited DePelchin's ability to develop the continuum as quickly as was hoped.

The first major services developed as alternatives to out-of-home care were the day treatment program and the home-based family preservation pro-gram. Both of these services were begun in 1983–84. The day treatment pro-gram was developed with a four-year, $400,000 foundation grant. The family preservation program was launched with a contract from the public child wel-fare agency and a United Way grant. As a result of these two services, agency staff working in both program divisions—child welfare and children's mental health—were able to maintain more children in their own homes while pro-viding services.

It became apparent that insurance companies would only pay for brief stays: fifteen to thirty days in the hospital, thirty to sixty days in residential treatment, and thirty to ninety days in day treatment. However, children often required more services in these programs. Consequently, the insurance companies were willing to pay for extensive outpatient services, even if the child and family received outpatient service for several months, because the cost was considerably less for these services than for substitute care.

In 1987 a large Houston-based health maintenance organization (HMO) with approximately 60,000 child and adolescent lives insured contacted DePelchin after a major hospital that had provided its child and adolescent inpatient psychiatric services terminated the contract. DePelchin Children's Center began providing psychiatric hospital services for this HMO in the summer of 1987, and discussions were initiated with the HMO regarding DePelchin's becoming the exclusive provider of its total mental health services to the 60,000 lives. Effective July 1, 1988, an agreement was entered into for DePelchin to be the exclusive provider of all mental health services with payment based on a discounted fee for service.

It was clear that the HMO expected most children and their families to be served on an outpatient basis. Until 1988, DePelchin Children's Center had a relatively small outpatient mental health service. DePelchin's management team obtained information from several major children's mental health organizations in the United States that had successfully used crisis intervention and other home-based interventions to reduce admissions to psychiatric hospitals. The information we obtained convinced us that we could duplicate the success of other organizations. DePelchin began to develop alternatives to out-of-home placements, and specifically to expand outpatient services. Consequently, this HMO contract was a major catalyst for DePelchin Children's Center to continue expanding its continuum of services, especially outpatient services.

Building Organizational Capacity

Following receipt of the first HMO contract, DePelchin management decided to explore ways to expand outpatient mental health service capacity. Most children and adolescents covered by this major HMO contract would only need outpatient services. We estimated an average of 500 weekly office therapy sessions would occur in this contract. Our pre-HMO service capacity was 250 weekly sessions. DePelchin Children's Center was already at capacity due to other contractual obligations.

DePelchin management considered two alternatives for increasing capacity of outpatient mental health services in order to successfully meet the HMO contract requirements. These alternatives were to develop the full continuum of care intraorganizationally or to do so through interorganizational arrangements. The initial decision was to expand internal capacity because of the very short time frame within which to respond to the projected increase in services. It was also important for DePelchin to successfully meet the performance expectations of the HMO. It was believed that the likelihood of meeting these expectations would be greatest if total control of operations was retained.

We initially planned to meet the requirements of the new HMO contact by using contract therapists. We realized, however, that this was not a viable long-term solution. We also needed additional office sites closer to the residences of the HMO subscribers.

Informal discussions concerning the possibility of merger occurred in 1987 between DePelchin Children's Center and Houston Child Guidance Center. The Child Guidance Center was a fifty-eight-year old children's mental health organization that had a good reputation in the Houston area. Management of the two organizations had identified some strategic advantage to a merger. Child Guidance lacked easy access to residential treatment and hospital services. DePelchin needed to expand its outpatient service delivery capacity.

Both boards were committed to their respective medical directors and chief executive officers. Merger discussions were terminated in early 1988 because of the boards' inability to agree on the selection of one individual to be the new chief executive officer and one individual to be the medical director of the combined organization.

Building an Interorganizational Continuum of Care

When it became apparent that DePelchin Children's Center could not expand outpatient service delivery capacity through a merger with Houston Child Guidance Center, management began exploring other options, including an alliance with the local children's hospital. Texas Children's Hospital was a training site for child psychiatry residents from Baylor College of Medicine. Although the hospital did not have a formal inpatient pediatric psychiatric service, it used psychiatric residents to provide consultation services to children who presented mental illness symptoms. The hospital and Baylor College of Medicine also jointly operated an outpatient mental health clinic for children and their families. The clinic was staffed by medical school faculty, psychiatric residents, psychology interns, and social work post-master's fellows. The clinic primarily served indigent clients. Only 20% of the clients paid for services through medical insurance benefits.

An alliance became desirable when the three parties realized that each organization brought capabilities and experiences to the alliance needed by the other two. Baylor brought experience and reputation as a training institution with considerable faculty expertise in treating mental illness. Texas Children's Hospital brought an outpatient mental health clinic and its reputation for serving the needs of children and adolescents. However, it lacked easy access to inpatient children's and adolescents' mental health services. DePelchin Children's Center brought an array of inpatient residential treatment and partial hospital services for children. It required access to and capacity for outpatient services.

Terms of the Agreement.   Three principles threaded through the alliance agreement: joint staff appointments, service unit integration, and procedural changes. In order to develop the alliance, DePelchin's medical director was appointed to three positions: chief of psychiatry at Baylor College of Medicine, medical director for DePelchin, and head of child psychiatry at Texas Children's Hospital. It was thought that this joint appointment would assure easy access to services and continuity of patient care for children at both Texas Children's Hospital and DePelchin Children's Center.

The clinic at the hospital was moved to the DePelchin Children's Center campus in late 1987 in order to integrate outpatient services with the other mental health services. Staff for the clinic continued to be composed of faculty and trainees from Baylor College of Medicine and DePelchin Children's Center staff.

Psychiatric residents were instructed to refer children and adolescents to DePelchin when they needed follow-up mental health services. Some referrals came through this process but they were far fewer than projected, and usually uninsured. It appeared that most insured children receiving psychiatric treatment at the hospital were engaged with a private psychiatrist when they entered. Frequently, a child's pediatrician had a relationship with a private child psychiatrist and referred to that practitioner. These private psychiatrists often had a preexisting affiliation with a for-profit psychiatric hospital system and referred child patients to that system.

The net outcome was too great an imbalance in the ratio of indigent clients to insured clients. The alliance, however, filled the outpatient capacity for DePelchin Children's Center's HMO clients.

Difficulties in the Alliance.   In 1991 key actors in the alliance had changed, thereby weakening the earlier commitments to its success. Baylor selected a new department head for psychiatry. Texas Children's Hospital had a new chief executive officer. A nationally renowned psychiatrist with expertise in services to children traumatized by abuse was jointly recruited by Baylor and the hospitals both to head psychiatric services at Children's and to develop a specialized service for sexually and physically abused children.

These changes resulted in reduced service coordination. Additionally, coordinating the training assignments and clinical decision making of psychiatric residents rotating through both organizations became more difficult. Conflicts in clinical treatment plans for children receiving services from the institutions became more frequent.

It was important for DePelchin to shift more of its service delivery capacity from residential treatment and psychiatric hospital services to outpatient services and partial hospitalization. The changes in private insurance mental health funding begun in 1985 had accelerated by 1991. Most insurance companies were not contracting with managed care organizations to manage mental health services. The result was closure of many psychiatric hospitals and for-profit residential treatment facilities in Houston, and throughout the United States. The Greater Houston Hospital Council reported that between 1988 and 1992 the number of psychiatric hospital beds decreased by 55%. Insured census in partial hospital services had declined by an average of 30%. DePelchin's insured census in hospital services had declined by 40% in populations other than those served by the capitated HMO contract. Because of DePelchin's endowment funds and large contribution base, the organization was able to manage these industry changes without suffering major financial losses. However, management realized that unless it reduced residential treatment and psychiatric hospital bed space, and increased outpatient capacity and services, major financial losses would occur.

Building an Intraorganizational Continuum of Care

Between 1987 and 1991, DePelchin Children's Center had relied primarily on the alliance with Baylor and Texas Children's Hospital to staff most of its outpatient clinics. As the relationship with the alliance partners changed, greater operational inefficiencies occurred in the outpatient mental health clinic. DePelchin Children's Center's cost per hour of therapy rose above market competition. Service volume did not increase as projected. Consequently, a decision was made in early 1991 by DePelchin management to consider other options for expanding outpatient service capacity and to reduce reliance on Baylor faculty and residents as clinic staff.

Simultaneously, Houston Child Guidance Center was being hurt by these market changes. It too had experienced a 30% drop in partial hospital service use. The management and board of Child Guidance were reviewing their options. In December 1991, a board member of Houston Child Guidance Center contacted a DePelchin board member indicating interest on the part of the Child Guidance in holding merger discussions with DePelchin.

Representatives of both boards and the two chief executive officers held two meetings between December 1991 and the end of January 1992 to explore the possibility of a merger. The numerous advantages of a merger of the two organizations quickly became apparent. A merger could enable DePelchin Children's Center to fulfill its mission of providing a full continuum of mental health and child welfare services to insured clients, public sector clients, and indigent clients. Child Guidance could easily access the various levels of out-of-home care provided by DePelchin. Economy of effort could be achieved by effectively combining the outpatient and partial hospital program of both organizations. Competition for managed care business could be reduced because both organizations held a number of managed care contracts. However, both organizations received significant United Way funding for provision of services to indigent people living in and around the Houston area.

Intensive discussions began in February 1992, and the merger was consummated effective April 1, 1992. The leadership of the combined boards supported the merger and the changes required to integrate the two organizations. The major issue that derailed the 1987 merger discussions, the roles of the respective medical and executive directors, was not present in 1992. Houston Child Guidance was without a full-time medical director, and the Child Guidance chief executive officer, a former banker, was informed that he would report to the DePelchin Children's Center chief executive officer.

The speed with which the merger was completed is attributable to financial losses being experienced by Houston Child Guidance Center. It had incurred losses of $500,000 on a budget of $4,000,000 during the first half of FY 1992. A delay would have resulted in greater financial losses to be covered by DePelchin. The rapidity of the merger made it impossible to adequately prepare staff of either organization for the changes associated with the merger. Child Guidance staff viewed the merger as a takeover; DePelchin staff viewed the use of DePelchin funds to cover Child Guidance's financial losses as a neglect of both staff salary increments and new program development. Conflicts occurred between the two staff groups and led to operation of separate divisions, one for mental health services and one for child welfare services for longer than management preferred.

Initially, all Child Guidance programs were maintained, although they were subject to ongoing review for clinical effectiveness and financial viability. The financial plan required across-the-board staff reductions in order to eliminate the operational deficit. Most of the staff reductions occurred from within the ranks of the Child Guidance employees.

The two organizations' outpatient services were operated separately. A transition team was assigned the responsibility of developing an integration time line. Child Guidance satellite offices were used immediately to provide services to DePelchin's managed care clients who could be more conveniently served at those offices. The two organizations' partial hospital programs operated separately until the end of the school year, when they were consolidated into one facility at the Child Guidance Center in summer 1992.

Progress was being made toward expansion of the continuum of care within the organization. The merger enabled DePelchin to significantly expand its outpatient mental health service capacity. During 1992 and 1993 several additional managed care contracts were signed. Several new school-based counseling programs were developed in partnership with local school districts. The home-based family preservation program was expanded with a new federal grant. DePelchin Children's Center had gained valuable experience in managing the capitated payment contract with the HMO that included 65,000 child and adolescent lives. A utilization management system had been developed. A client satisfaction survey process had been implemented. However, additional changes needed to be made.

Organizational Restructuring to Enhance Service Operations

DePelchin needed to be administratively and programmatically restructured to become more financially efficient, and to more efficiently and effectively deliver services. DePelchin experienced financial losses in both 1992 and 1993 in the range of $200,000 on a budget in excess of $16,000,000. The agency's expenses were too high and lengths of stay in residential treatment and psychiatric hospital services were too long in comparison to the managed behavioral health care industry in greater Houston. Although the losses wee manageable, it was clear that greater losses would occur unless changes were made.

Initial changes focused on fiscal operations. DePelchin's business office lacked the experience and proficiency to manage copayment collections and the required follow-up tracking of insurance claims that had not been paid or had been only partially paid. The result was a significant increase in insurance receivables some of which were never collected and later had to be written off.

The experience of running losses in two consecutive years and the frequent delays in receiving payments from managed care organizations necessitated improved case management. A plan was developed, and subsequently adopted, to increase unrestricted cash reserves that could be used to assume risk in capitated payment contracts, to develop new programs, and to fund cash flow. Cash reserves were increased to $700,000 by allocating funds from bequests to the unrestricted fund rather than to the endowment fund.

The deficits convinced us that we also needed to devote more staff resources to managing client service utilization. Many staff members continued to wrestle with such issues as length of stay, utilization management, outside case reviews, and decision making by managed care companies. One of the major challenges for DePelchin was undoing the mind-set many clinicians acquired in graduate training, which frequently focuses on longer term psychodynamic treatment. Their training runs counter to the realities of providing services under managed care, which emphasizes solution-focused, brief treatment.

In 1993, a utilization manager was employed by DePelchin Children's Center. Prior to this hiring, a committee process was used for utilization review. The individual employed was given the responsibility to train staff, interface with managed care companies, and review all cases that exceeded expected lengths of treatment according to both industry standards and norms developed by a staff committee. This new utilization management process contributed significantly to reduced lengths of treatment. The focus on utilization management, as well as improved business office operations, increased profitability. DePelchin ended 1994 with revenue in excess of expenditures of $150,000, and a surplus of $350,000 was achieved for 1995.

Finally, it became apparent that DePelchin Children's Center needed to operationally restructure from two programmatic divisions, one for child welfare and one for mental health services, into a single programmatic division organized around service groups. Increasingly, managed care organizations were willing to authorize and reimburse for some traditional child welfare services targeted to treatment of behavioral health problems. These services were home-based therapy, treatment foster family care, and emergency shelter service. These services were operated out of DePelchin's child welfare division and needed to be combined with outpatient mental health services and day treatment services, which were provided out of the agency's mental health division. Each program division had its own assessment process and administrative structures. Not only was this duplicative and costly, but it was also difficult for each division to access services offered by the other division.

The restructuring resulted in all services being organized under one chief operating officer for programs. Management carefully assessed each service in terms of treatment philosophy, goals, and client populations. Based on the findings, programs were grouped together into service groups. All residential programs, including the emergency shelters, were placed in a single service group. All outpatient or home-based counseling programs were grouped together. These changes were necessary to achieve financial savings by reducing the number of supervisory and administrative positions and to bring integration to the service delivery system.

Change in the Operational Environment

By 1995, behavioral health care provided by private insurance was predominantly delivered through managed care systems. In Houston, more than 70% of all insured individuals were receiving their behavioral health care coverage through managed care organizations. DePelchin's management team concluded that public systems would also move toward managed care models of payment and service delivery. Texas Senate Bill 10 mandating statewide implementation of managed care for Medicaid, including behavioral health care, passed in the 1995 legislative session. The state agencies providing child protective services and mental health services also had task forces developing plans for managed care delivery systems.

At the same time, DePelchin negotiated a new contract that incorporated some managed care principles with the county mental health authority. For the first time, case management responsibilities for clients referred by the public mental health authority were transferred to DePelchin. The contract contained sufficient flexibility that DePelchin could move a child across programs as needed as long as total expenditures for the expected number of children to be served stayed within contract limits. Financial incentives were provided in the contract to use less restrictive services when these services were appropriate.

DISCUSSION AND IMPLICATIONS FOR PRACTICE

By its definition, managed care is a system of care delivery that influences utilization, contains costs of services, and measures performance. As managed care continues to evolve, and as it becomes the predominant service delivery model, children's agencies should anticipate a range of challenges. These will occur in delivery system structures, quality control of services, and development of preventive and early intervention programs.

Organizations will be required to consider the advantages and disadvantages of developing capacity internally or by participating in networks or alliances with other organizations. In most cases, small to medium-sized agencies will not be able to participate in public and private managed care service delivery unless they align with other agencies. Some large agencies, such as DePelchin, may be able to continue to secure public sector contracts without aligning with others, but there is political risk in this strategy. For example, the State of Kansas signed contracts with one organization in each region to provide all out-of-home care for the child welfare population but awarded all contracts to organizations that included other service providers in their systems of care.

The trend seems clear that managed care organizations are increasingly purchasing services from large provider organizations or networks of providers. For example, the Texas Medicaid Managed Care Plan used large HMOs to manage all services: medical, surgical, and behavioral health. Usually, the HMO subcontracts the behavioral health services to a managed care company that then turns around and attempts to contract with a network or alliance of providers rather than multiple individual providers. Contracting with a network or alliance of providers is more efficient for the managed care organization. Too few states have implemented managed care models for child welfare for definitive trends to be identified. However, in states where such a model has been introduced, such as Tennessee and Kansas, network or alliance development has been common.

In the future, children's agencies can expect to encounter service delivery models that utilize at-risk arrangements whereby providers are penalized financially for providing too many days of the most expensive, out-of-home care. Providers will be expected to serve more children and families with outpatient or home-based services and will be penalized financially if this does not occur at expected levels. Contractual arrangements will also become increasingly performance oriented. A focus on successful outcomes measured in terms of children improving in behavior, school performance, and family functioning will become prevalent.

Children's agencies will need to become more knowledgeable about and to implement quality control systems. These new systems will not replace the traditional mechanism, the supervisory conference, but they will reshape the mix of quality control techniques. Management information systems that support clinicians and enable organizations to measure clinician-specific quality will become essential. As the transition to more sophisticated management information systems occurs, nonprofit children's agencies will need to reassess the traditional supervisory structures typically in place in agencies. It is not necessary, nor is it affordable, to provide weekly supervision to highly trained clinicians.

A method many children's agencies are using to assure high-quality staff and high-quality performance in a highly efficient environment is the use of professional credentialing. Credentialing is the process by which an organization determines the graduate training, postgraduate experience, and successful clinical outcomes required of each clinician for each specific clinical service provided. Recredentialing of staff to provide services is based on measuring employee performance against expected outcomes, using the organization's quality improvement and utilization management systems. This approach to managing clinical staff should result in greater controls over costs and encourage staff to take more responsibility for their professional growth and development. The result should be increased efficiencies that are necessary for nonprofit organizations to compete successfully with for-profit organizations.

Managed care organizations have been slow to purchase programs and services that prevent the onset of mental health problems. There will be gradual increases in funding for preventive services by managed care organizations as providers become more competent at demonstrating the cost savings associated with prevention efforts in mental health services.

Several states now provide funding for a primary prevention of child abuse project, Healthy Families America. In 1996, several large Houston area foundations announced a major collaborative effort in which more than $10,000,000 over five years will be granted to agencies working together to prevent children's mental illness, child abuse, and school failure. The success or failure of prevention efforts such as these will be an important determinant of the availability of new funds for preventive work.

In the late 1980s, DePelchin Children's Center began placing greater emphasis on managed care and therefore has viewed it as necessary and consistent with the organization's mission and vision. It has been our experience that most managed care systems purchase reasonable services at reasonable rates, thereby reducing excessive inpatient utilization and encouraging development of innovative, less restrictive treatment methods. In Houston, between 1985 and 1990, days of psychiatric hospitalization per 1,000 lives declined by 50% to 60%. Some insurance companies began contracting with service providers to provide mobile crisis services and "twenty-three-hour admissions" in order to avoid unnecessary hospitalization of children; that it, hospitals and residential treatment facilities are paid $600 to $800 per service to provide observation, supervision, and intense therapy.

DePelchin's experiences with private managed care has stimulated the agency to develop values and systems that allow managed care principles to be applied to public sector contracts. Experience gained in developing and operating utilization management and review systems based on clinical protocols have been adapted to guide placement decisions for the public child welfare population. The tracking of costs by client and by unit of service, learned under private managed care, will be important in successfully managing public sector managed care contracts.

CHAPTER 9

Organizational Reform in a Community Mental Health Center

Stephen Christian-Michaels
Chief Operating Officer,
Family Services of Western Pennsylvania, Pittsburgh

Gary Noll
Director, Behavioral and Mental Health Services,
DuPage County Health Department

Stephen P. Wernet
Professor, School of Social Service,
Saint Louis University

Community mental health agencies have increased their involvement in managed care activities. The change seems to be driven by the desire to secure additional revenue by attracting new business. Also driving the change is the shift by public funding sources to the use of managed care approaches. These public funders are converting from grants and fee-for-service payment systems to funding streams that emphasize increased accountability and cost containment.

This chapter focuses on one community mental health agency's strategy to use the shift to managed care approaches to reform its delivery system. Furthermore, it reports on the impact of managed care on the access, efficiency, and deflection outcomes in a public mental health center. The application of managed care concepts allowed DuPage County Health Department's Behavioral and Mental Health Services to reform its operation and thereby better serve the population of adults with severe and persistent mental illness and children with serious emotional disturbance. This reform occurred in an envi-

The authors thank Bill Coats for his conceptual contribution to this chapter. His ability to see the larger picture helped in its writing, as well as in the reform it describes.

ronment of increasing costs and increasing population with no proportional growth in public funding for services.

The specific managed care concepts relied on most heavily were gate-keeping, utilization management, and utilization review. Gatekeeping is addressed by the creation of central assessment for most clients, by clarity of admission criteria, and by reducing or eliminating the time between admission into the system and delivery of service. Regulating the type of service and its duration, with special attention to deflection from hospitalization, exemplifies the implementation of utilization management.

Organizational reform was carried out by 1) asserting control over a system of care that had a poor track record of accountability, 2) redesigning the system of care using managed care principles, and 3) selling the reform to internal and external stakeholders. A secondary theme that runs through this account is the difficulty of operating a mission-driven organization that resides in, and is part of, a governmental structure yet challenged by a changing marketplace.

ORGANIZATIONAL CONTEXT

Behavioral and Mental Health Services of the DuPage County Health Department provides community mental health services in a county of 888,000 residents. DuPage County is a fast-growing suburban area in northern Illinois. It has realized growth of 42% in the past seventeen years. It is the second largest populated county in Illinois, exceeded only by Cook County, which includes urban Chicago. DuPage County is made up of thirty-seven municipalities with forty-eight school districts. The county encompasses five hundred square miles—twenty miles by twenty-five miles.

More than three thousand clients are served annually through a full range of crisis, assessment, assertive case management/home-based services, counseling, day treatment, and residential services. Brief crisis services are provided to another 750 individuals. Behavioral and Mental Health Services static capacity, that is, the total number of the clients served at a particular point in time, is 2,200. Dynamic capacity, that is, the annual flow of clients through the system, averages 3,200 clients.

Over the past fifteen years, the population served has become more severely impaired. One of the central admission criteria to enter the system for clinical services is a Global Assessment of Functioning (GAF) score of 50 or less. This measure of functioning is based on the therapist's assessment of the client's level of functioning using anchor descriptions of behavior that are associated with a 100-point scale. The GAF is the measure used in Axis 5 of the multiaxial diagnostic system. *Diagnostic and Statistical Manual of Mental Disorders, Fourth Edition* (American Psychiatric Association, 1994). The GAF was modified from the Global Assessment Scale (Endicott, Spritzer, Fleiss, & Coehn, 1976). GAF scores are not used as an entrance criterion to crisis services because these services are provided to a broader population. However, crisis care is brief and time limited. Psychoeducational services are provided to individuals with higher levels of functioning as a preventive or risk reduction strategy.

Behavioral and Mental Health Services is staffed by 176 full-time employees, 154 part-time employees, and 5 full-time-equivalent psychiatrists. Its operating budget is nearly $14 million. Approximately half of the budget is state funded; the remainder is generated through local property taxes.

Behavioral and Mental Health Services is a community mental health agency embedded in a county health department. This has advantages as well as disadvantages. With nearly half of the annual budget derived from local sources, Services has been somewhat insulated from the impact of both the state's uneven planning efforts and its funding fluctuations. The Illinois Department of Human Services Office of Mental Health has targeted its resources to the most impaired population. The mission of Behavioral and Mental Health Services is consistent with that of the state mental health authority but incongruous with that of its host organization, the DuPage County Health Department. The Health Department's Community Health Services and Environmental Health Services adopts a public health perspective that emphasizes primary and secondary prevention strategies, while Behavioral and Mental Health Services focuses 97% of its resources on tertiary care.

The Illinois mental health delivery system is a state-administered system that includes eleven state psychiatric hospitals. Local community mental health agencies are funded primarily through grants and Medicaid reimbursed fee-for-services. Medicaid funding for community mental health centers was only established in 1990. Torrey and Wolfe (1990) ranked Illinois forty-fourth out of fifty states in per capita funding on mental health services. This situation exists despite Illinois' status as twelfth in per capita income. Illinois is ranked thirty-first compared to the other states in terms of overall system effectiveness.

Like many other states, Illinois had begun pursuing a Medicaid waiver for a managed care model in its publicly funded health care system. However, because the Federal Omnibus Reconciliation Act of 1997 increased states' ability to shift their Medicaid funds to a managed care funding stream, Illinois had dropped its waiver application. The original application would have carved out behavioral health services. The current plan for managed Medicaid is an expansion of the voluntary health maintenance organization (HMO) enrollment program beyond Cook County to Medicaid recipients who receive a monthly cash grant and Medicaid health coverage (medical assistance and grant) and are part of the welfare reform initiative, that is, temporary assistance to needy families. Medicaid recipients who only have Medicaid health coverage (medical assistance—no grant) will be phased in through voluntary enrollment in late 1998. Within two years, the majority of Medicaid recipients are likely to be involuntarily enrolled in HMOs, with a few excluded populations. The current HMO contracts are written so that behavioral health services are carved in. Community mental health centers are being encouraged to contract with the HMOs as subcontracted behavioral health care providers. It is uncertain what the impact of managed Medicaid will be on behavioral health care services. Depending on how it is implemented, managed Medicaid could either improve or worsen the effectiveness of behavioral health care.

In Illinois attempts at mental health system reform have produced a series of incomplete initiatives that reflect lack of popular support for services for the mentally ill. One serious deficiency of the system is the disconnection between state psychiatric hospitals and community mental health centers. They are two separate systems of care with different funding streams. There has been little statewide incentive to reduce the reliance on inpatient care and shift to greater community support. When adult clients were deinstitutionalized during the 1950s and 1960s, nursing homes rather than group homes became the alternative residual care system. In 1989 the Illinois Department of Mental Health and Developmental Disabilities implemented a statewide gatekeeping system and home-based services for children. This ultimately led to the closure of all state hospital beds for children and adolescents in the seven counties that constitute the Chicago metropolitan area. Unfortunately, this type of systemic response has not been applied to the adult care system. The summary of the 1990 Torrey report for Illinois was: "Going nowhere fast."

PROBLEMS WITHIN THE COMMUNITY MENTAL HEALTH SYSTEM

The community mental health movement was created to overcome problems evident in the institutional treatment of individuals with mental illness. While the principles of community mental health address the limitations of institutional care, too often community mental health centers have been unable to cope with the breadth of problems presented by these individuals. There are several reasons for these failures. First, funding has not followed clients into the community. Community mental health centers have been increasingly expected to serve individuals with mental illness but without concomitant increases in or reallocation of resources for these services.

Second, with inadequate resources, community mental health centers typically have long waiting lists. Clients can wait months to start treatment while other, higher functioning clients receive services for an extended period of time.

Third, community managed health centers have frequently neither identified nor linked into a system of care either adults with severe and persistent mental illness or children with serious emotional disturbance. Community mental health centers tend to use office based, individual modes of treatment, which are easy to administer and more comfortable and satisfying for staff, rather than other treatment modalities—for example, group treatment, home-based treatment, assertive case management, mobile assessment, and crisis intervention—with proven success in treating individuals with serious and persistent mental illness. Therefore, these centers are serving higher functioning clients in a predominantly clinic-based delivery system.

Fourth, a remnant of patient blaming survives. The client is treated in a condescending manner rather than as a partner in treatment focused on strengths.

Fifth, high-risk clients with severe symptoms, violent behavior, or dual diagnoses (mental illness and substance abuse) have not been adequately retained in treatment programs and experience discontinuous episodes of treatment. Too often funding sources and staff education contribute to fragmentation of services into the specialty fields of mental health, substance abuse treatment, and criminal justice. This compartmentalization circumvents the needs of high-risk, multisymptom and dually diagnosed individuals thereby frustrating both clients and staff.

Sixth, like much of the health care system today, the public mental health delivery system is evaluated on the volume of services rendered, with more being better, rather than on outcome measures of effectiveness. This perspective permeates evaluation of agencies, teams, and individual staff members.

Finally, accountability is absent. Treatment tends to be undefined and is provided behind closed doors in isolation from other team members. Confidentiality has frequently been invoked to protect the therapist from being held accountable. Evaluation of agency outcomes was also avoided with the excuse that measurement of change in this field is too difficult or impossible. With the lack of measurable outcomes, little wonder that the field suffers from a lack of public understanding or support.

PRINCIPLES FOR REFORMING A SYSTEM

Management innovations are frequently transferred from the private sector to the public sector and implemented in narrowly defined initiatives that serve only a small subpopulation or focus only on the financing of the system. Innovations such as zero-based budgeting, continuous quality improvement, total quality management, and management by objectives are often adopted by the public sector with insufficient understanding of the technology and are only partly implemented with no adaptation to the needs of a public care system. The current interest in managed care may be another example of this problem. Managed care, if treated as a set of discrete techniques, will not control escalating mental health costs.

To improve the system of care, the principles of managed care need to be used to support the mission of a community mental health agency or a larger mental health system of care. Key principles of community mental health must be kept in mind as the overriding structure in any and every reform. These principles include accessibility, least restrictive level of care, continuity of care, efficiency, and community ownership. Managed care in a public mental health system "involves the organization of an accessible and accountable service delivery system that is designed to consolidate and flexibly deploy resources so as to provide comprehensive, continuous, cost-efficient and effective mental health services to targeted individuals in their home communities" (Hoge, Davidson, Griffith, Sledge, & Howenstine, 1994, p. 1087). The synthesis of managed care principles and community mental health are expected to produce the following outcomes:

Increased accessibility to services

Decreased reliance on inpatient/residential care via gatekeeping

Deflection and use of a continuum of care that matches levels of need with levels of care

Clearly defined sets of intervention into service packages or "bundles"

Increased efficiency due to utilization review, utilization management, and the use of clinical protocols that rationalize allocation decisions

Increased focus on treating chronic conditions through disease management through case management and other long-term supportive services with less reliance on acute episodic care

Improved quality as reflected through greater customer satisfaction

Enhancement of both outcome indicators and process indicators to drive quality improvement and continuous system redesign

Improved community functioning through community ownership, community involvement, and community development

Several perspectives or assumptions should support systemic change and diffusion of innovative technology into any large organization, especially a public sector bureaucracy.

Recognition That the System Is Faulty

Too often individual members of a system, whether staff, programs, or entire agencies, are blamed for systemic inadequacies. The problem is the system, not the staff, not the programs, not the finances—the system. To institute reforms, leadership of an agency must assume responsibility for correcting the ineffectiveness of the system while trying to minimize the blame that tends to be projected onto individuals and programs. When Behavioral and Mental Health Services introduced a new alternative to inpatient adult care, a mobile intensive case management unit, the admitting staff were commended for their past successes while the system's weaknesses in alternative care were identified. This alternative to inpatient adult care was introduced as a way to deflect the seriously and persistently mentally ill from hospitalization.

Change Planned with the Population in Mind

Serving a population requires agency leadership to plan and prioritize in a very conscious manner. The majority of children and adolescents admitted to the state hospital generally had not received any services from the Behavioral and Mental Health Services. Between 1980 and 1985 Services retrained its staff and publicized its specialty with children and adolescents who have severe emotional disturbance. The agency then began to refer the lower risk population to other agencies. It required a conscious decision and a consistent focus to make this shift to examining and prioritizing the needs of the whole population. This change also made it possible for us to get closer to realizing our mission of serving only persons with severe and persistent mental illness or serious emotional disturbance.

Change as Nonlinear, Multicausal, Multilevel Intervention

Systemic change can only be achieved incrementally and only as subsets of the system succeed. To change a system, subsystems thought to be amenable to change must be either identified or incubated. Islands of excellence as laboratories of change can then be established. We chose to incubate a new culture by constituting new programs with new staff and housing them away from the rest of the system. As these programs evolved a new culture they created new performance norms or expectations for excellence in patient care.

For example, as an intensive set of alternative services to inpatient care, home-based children's services were purposely developed outside the milieu of the outpatient clinic in order to establish a new set of norms and expectations. The culture of proactive case managers began to expand beyond the children's outreach program to other children's services and is now being expanded into adult services. Another incubated program was the women's substance abuse program, which was developed off site. This island of excellence generated great staff excitement, radically different ways of delivering services, and a significant decrease in the number of toxic births for substance-abusing mothers. Had either of these programs been housed in the traditional system, the powerful effect of group norms would likely have minimized the development of these innovative programs.

The next challenge is to integrate the new culture into the rest of the system thereby changing the larger system over time. Changing one part of the system will change the larger system, but forethought must be given to channeling the change. For example, outpatient staff is now providing more home-based services; similar to the work of children services, adult services are beginning to use wraparound funds to support clients; reducing adult admissions has become a much higher priority than in the past in the adult service subsystem.

Any change to the delivery system will set up the conditions in the next required reform. Centralizing alcoholism services to one site sets up the conditions to also centralize office-based child and adolescent services and, to a lesser degree, office-based adult services. This move from generalist focus to specialist focus creates the need for a generalist approach in the years to come, as the pendulum swings too far to a specialist focus.

APPLYING MANAGED CARE PRINCIPLES TO REFORM A MENTAL HEALTH SYSTEM

Table 1 summarizes managed care principles, problems related to not meeting our mission, and solutions generated to overcome systemic problems. The goal of the reform was to determine who needed what care, at what level, and to deliver that care quickly, effectively, and efficiently. The process of reform had three elements: taking control of a system with little accountability to clients or taxpayers, redesigning a system of care, and selling the reform to internal and external stakeholders. This reform occurred over fifteen years. The reform is incremental, a work-in-progress, and continues today. Creating a match between organizational vision and operation did not occur throughout the entire system nor was it fully embraced by all staff.

Accessibility

Behavioral and Mental Health Services evolved into a system with multiple sites and programs and many points of access. Waiting times to access services lengthened. High-risk clients were often not following through on discharge plans from hospitals.

A reengineering approach was taken with middle managers and direct care staff of the various front-door-type services. With the development of a crisis intervention program, one systemwide access point was developed and implemented for individuals in crisis. The problem was that potential clients and referral sources would have to determine whether or not they were in crisis. Nonemergency intake services were only available between 8:30 A.M. and 4:30 P.M., five days a week. However, over a period of three months access crisis services were redesigned. Five months later a single phone number for crisis and admission for the system was widely advertised. This element extended the hours of nonemergency outpatient admissions to twenty-four hours a day, seven days a week. From the gains in new efficiencies, freed-up resources were used to create a utilization management team. This team's functions are described in a later section.

Another accessibility innovation was combining mental health assessment with psychiatric evaluation. In the past, the process of serving most public mental health clients resulted in their waiting a prolonged time for services, and the clients most at risk were likely to deteriorate. An intake worker

Managed Care Principles Used to Drive Reform

Managed Care Principles	Problems	Solutions
Accessibility	14 Access points to service	Created single entry point
	Wait for assessment	Centralized assessment
	Wait for psychiatric evaluation	Combined evaluations
	Not attracting high-risk clients	Outreach services
Gatekeeping	Reliance on expensive restrictive care	Assessors/gatekeepers
	Inability to titrate care	Length-of-stay authorization
		Authorize number of sessions
		Treatment packages formalize criteria
Comprehensive continuum	Lack of internal treatment capacity	Alternative services to inpatient care
	Lack of intensive services	3 treatment arrays with levels of care
	Inefficient treatment modalities	Extended case management
		Group homes and apartments
		Medication groups
		Group therapy increased
		Psychoeducation classes
		Home-based treatment developed
Disease management	Not retaining high-risk clients	No-close policy for severe and persistently mentally ill clients
Utilization management	Consumption-oriented incentives	Shift to treatment by teams
	Interminable treatment	Shift to team evaluations
	Inadequate documentation of service	Shift focus to outcomes
		Institute peer evaluations
		Limit on length of stay
		Reauthorization/appeals
		Record reviews
		Concurrent reviews

assigned each client to a therapist who both conducted the evaluation and ultimately provided most of the services. Each therapist evaluated her or his own clients, decided whether the client needed a psychiatric evaluation, and if necessary scheduled the evaluation, perhaps a month after the client entered the system. This procedure meant a delay in treatment and frequently a mismatch between the diagnosis and treatment plans of the therapist and the psychiatrist.

Under the system reform, a central assessment team was created. The assessment function was centralized from as many as seven sites to one site, and from as many as fifty assessors to seven. This change reduced the waiting time for assessment and treatment and helped to systematize who was admitted to the agency. It generated comprehensive assessments with unified diagnosis and treatment plans. Medication regimes could start after the first appointment without delay. Working as a team, the assessor and psychiatrist each contributed a unique perspective and developed a holistic assessment.

Centralization shortened the time that clients waited for both assessment and treatment and improved the quality of the assessments. Record compliance also increased dramatically because assessment was centralized.

Outreach services were created to help link high-risk clients to existing services. Liaison case management staff was assigned to public and private psychiatric hospitals to identify clients who met the agency's admission criteria. Services included discharge planning, aftercare groups, crisis intervention, psychiatric evaluations, medication monitoring, and case management until clients are stabilized and linked into less intensive outpatient services. These services were so successful that four private psychiatric hospitals now purchase them to serve the population most at risk.

Gatekeeping

A key redesign element was the gatekeeping components that were put into place. This involved the institution of more control over how clients entered the system, how they were assigned to various levels of care, and how treatment episodes were reauthorized. Assessors in the centralized assessment team are now asked to provide two functions for the delivery system: diagnostic evaluation and gatekeeping.

The central assessment program was instituted initially for adults with serious mental illness and later expanded to substance abuse and children. The process of centralizing assessment involved, first, selected therapists at each site to conduct assessments and, second, common staffing once a week to make clinical dispositions. While cumbersome and time consuming, the process helped win staff acceptance of the change. Ultimately, whole staff positions were allocated to a new assessment unit. This process allowed staff to both adjust to a system in which the assessor is the gatekeeper and retool for other roles and responsibilities within the system.

Once the client's level of functioning, clinical diagnosis, and clinical needs have been evaluated, the assessor then decides whether the client meets the entrance criteria by reviewing the initial admission screening. The assessor decides what level of care is required and orders one or several treatment services bundled into treatment packages with a length of stay. In the future, this authorization may also include a specific number of sessions.

Given the stagnant funding for mental health services and the rapid population growth in DuPage County, Behavioral and Mental Health Services was forced to deal with allocation decisions and rationing of services before other mental health systems faced this dilemma. The methods employed involved 1) narrowing the criteria to be accepted for a diagnostic evaluation, 2) raising the threshold for admission for treatment services in terms of level of functioning, 3) reducing the initial length of stay before reauthorization is required, 4) limiting initial authorization for each ordered service, and 5) requiring reauthorization from the program supervisor for ongoing treatment.

Part of the challenge of distributing resources equally meant creating unambiguous entrance criteria for clinical services provided by Behavioral and Mental Health Services. Admission criteria were established for emergency services and for assessment services. These criteria are narrow, given the limited resources available. Listed below are the criteria for an adult assessment:

1. Discharge from hospital/residential treatment center and need aftercare service, or

2. Major mental disorder present with or without substance abuse that if not treated will result in a severe loss in functioning and therefore needs acute care as defined by emergency service criteria, and

3. Has completed an episode of treatment with Behavioral and Mental Health Services access crisis services, or with Behavioral and Mental Health Services outpatient services, or with other community counseling agencies, or

4. Other community based service provider refers because they no longer can provide the intensity of services required to prevent hospitalization or extrusion from the home and are willing to provide joint treatment planning with Behavioral and Mental Health Services staff.

These above criteria made it possible to ration services to those needing them most, but based on a rational set of rules. The criteria for educational/support group services and crisis services were much less narrow, making it possible to serve a large number of people for very brief episodes of care.

Another gatekeeping function is the service provided by the agency to state psychiatric hospitals. All clients requesting inpatient care at a state psychiatric hospital are screened and assessed to assure that only those who require that level of care are sent to the hospital. Intensive services are provided as an alternative to inpatient care for those who might otherwise be admitted to the hospital. Alternative services range from short-term respite center for adults and in-home respite services for children and adolescents to in-home therapy, case management, and wraparound funds to purchase goods and services to reduce the need to extrude the client from the family and community. These services are often provided for as much as twenty hours of quick services within the first week with the intent of wrapping clients with services that they might otherwise have received in institutional care but can now receive in the community at a lower cost.

Comprehensive Continuum

Over ten years Behavioral and Mental Health Services was redesigned from a counseling clinic to an integrated system offering a comprehensive continuum of care. The agency specialized in treating the highest risk clientele and had the lowest rate of hospitalization for children and adults in state psychiatric hospitals in the metropolitan region. The intent was to shift clients from long-term individual therapy to group treatment, medication groups, socialization/recreational activities, and psychoeducational services. Specialized educational classes were also developed for clients and their families. Intensive in-home services were used as an alternative to inpatient care when office-based services were not intensive enough to meet the needs of the client. Mobile services included outreach case management, off-site emergency assessments, assertive case management, in-home therapy, and respite services. Crisis intervention, crisis respite beds, sustaining care case management, and residential group homes/apartment programs all acted as supportive services to a population with severe and persistent mental illness.

Services were redesigned, breaking down the distinctions between the thirty-six different programs, and reorganized into three arrays of care: assessment, adult, and child and adolescent arrays. Levels of care were nested within each of the three arrays. They varied as follows:

Risk reduction prevention

Low risk (referral to counseling agencies or private practitioners)

Intermediate care

Extended care (sustaining care)

Acute care (emergency and crisis services)

Inpatient care

The current initiative is to further delineate the level of care between intermediate care and extended care. Clusters of treatment services are nested within each level of care in decreasing levels of intensity (intermediate care—

psychiatric visits only to twenty-four-hour transitional residential services). Each level of care has broad admission criteria including the GAF (Endicott et al., 1976) for adults and the Children's Global Assessment Scale (Shaffer et al., 1983). These measures of functioning are based on therapist assessment of the client's level of functioning using anchor behavioral descriptions that are associated with a 1 to 100 point scale. Level-of-functioning criteria for each level of care overlap because other criteria, such as social support, can offset severe disabilities; for example, level 2 GAF scores range between 35 and 50, while level 3 GAF scores range from 25 to 40. Other criteria for a level of care include capacity to maintain self after episode of treatment (level 2), multiple hospitalizations (level 3), and inability to care for self or others (level 5). An example array, the adult array, is displayed in figure 1.

A cluster of services is bundled together, such as counseling, case management, and crisis intervention. The bundle is called a treatment package. Each treatment package includes the following:

A brief description

Admission criteria

Exclusion criteria

Exit criteria

Length of stay

A list of billable services with the initial standard authorization

Weekly intensity of services

Maximum number of units

Average number of units

Maximum cost

Average cost

Qualification of staff delivering each billable service

The arrays and the treatment package descriptions were compiled into a treatment package manual (DuPage County Health Department, 1997). These arrays and treatment packages attempt to rationalize what had been a very complex and unorganized system of care.

Disease Management

The problem of retaining high-risk clients once they have been linked to community services is often overlooked, particularly if there is a long waiting list for services. Weekly outpatient therapy was not valued by this clientele, nor was it effective, and the therapist did not want to provide case management and other sustaining care services. It was necessary early in the reform process to confront both the passive method whereby high-risk clients were

FIGURE 1   Array of Adult Treatment Packages

LEVEL 0 RISK REDUCTION GAF OVER 50	LEVEL 2 INTERMEDIATE CARE GAF 35-50	LEVEL 3 EXTENDED CARE GAF 25-45	LEVEL 4 ACUTE CARE GAF 15-35	LEVEL 5 HOSPITAL CARE GAF 0-25
COPING SKILLS FOR FAMILIES 10 Weeks A-0-140	BASIC PSYCHIATRIC A-2-100	PSYCHIATRIC A-3-100	CRISIS COUNSELING A-4-100	AFTERCARE LINKAGE CASE MGT A-5-100
FREEDOM FROM FEAR 8 Weeks A-0-150	MEDICATION ADMIN. A-2-105	MEDICATION ADMIN. A-3-105	CRISIS PSYCHIATRIC A-4-110	ACUTE EMERG. PSYCH. SERVICES W/CASE MGT A-5-150
FAMILY SUPPORT GRP. ONGOING A-0-160	EDUCATION GROUPS A-2-110	MEDICATION GROUP A-3-110	CRISIS HOME CARE A-4-120	
SOUNDING BOARD ONGOING A-0-165	PRE-GRP COUNSELING A-2-115	BENEFIT COORDINATION CONSULTATION A-3-115	BENEFIT COORDIN. A-4-125	
EMOTIONAL INTENSITY FAMILY SUPPORT GROUP ONGOING A-0-170	MOOD DISORDER/ANXIETY SPECIALITY GROUP A-2-120	YOUNG ADULT CLINIC A-3-120	ADULT AFTERCARE A-4-130	
DUAL DX FAMILY SUPPORT GRP A-0-175	BRIEF COUNSELING A-2-130	OLDER ADULT CASE MGT A-3-130	INTENSIVE CASE MGT. A-4-200	
INFANT MENTAL HEALTH PARENT & CHILD PREV. 6 MONTHS A-0-180	CASE MANAGEMENT A-2-140	OLDER ADULT CLINIC A-3-140	INTENSIVE OUTPT. A-4-205	
	FAMILY COUNSELING A-2-150	DUAL DX MEDICATION (ONLY) CLINIC A-3-150		
	GROUP COUNSELING SERVICES 1-2-160	CLOZARIL CLINIC A-3-160	RESPITE CENTER A-4-500	
	INDIV. COUNSELING A-2-200	CHRONIC MEDICAL/PSYCH ILLNESS GROUP A-3-170	PARTIAL HOSPITAL. A-4-510	
	EMOT. INTENS. CLINIC A-2-210	DUAL RECOVERY IDENT. GRP, A-3-180		
	INFANT MENTAL HEALTH PARENTS W/AXIS 1 DX A-2-220	OSCAR GROUP A-3-190		
	WOMEN'S PROGRAM A-2-230	EMOT. ITENSITY GROUP COUNSELING A-3-200		
	SPECIALIZED WOMEN'S SERVICES A-2-240	DUAL RECOVERY SUPPORT GROUP A-3-210		
	PSYCH. SOCIAL REHAB. VOCATION PLACEMENT A-2-300	EXTENDED SUPPORT EMPLOYMENT A-3-220		
	INTERMITT. RESIDENT. A-2-400	INFANT MH-EXTENDED CARE A-3-230		
	24 HOUR CARE A-2-500	CASE MANAGEMENT EXTENDED A-3-240		
		EXTENDED TRANSITIONAL SERVICES A-3-300		
		ASSERTIVE COMM TX A-3-350		
		INTERMITTENT RESIDEN. CARE-EXTENDED A-3-400		
		24 HOUR RESIDENTIAL CARE-EXTENDED A-3-500		

leaving the system of care and the absence of aggressive outreach of specialized services to meet their needs. A disease management approach is essential to best serve the clients and manage limited resources. A "no-close" policy sent a clear message that the therapist was responsible for clients over a long period of time. However, because of the no-close policy, a dynamic tension was established with the service-rationing assumption that underlies utilization management.

With this message sent, an extended care level of services blossomed. Sustaining care case management is a less intense level of care, where intermittent supportive services are provided over a long duration. Less intensive case management, recreational services, drop-in socialization services, and vocational services are provided. Residential services such as group homes, transitional apartment programs, or clustered apartment programs provide the supportive services that sustain people with serious impairments. However, treatment protocols based on disease management require further development in order to proactively meet the needs of clients over their lifetimes.

Utilization Management

In a system, the therapist implements the organization's or program's policies regarding length of stay, who stays in treatment, and who is discharged. Some adult clients with severe and persistent mental illness leave treatment through what is perceived as lack of commitment or resistance to treatment. At Behavioral and Mental Health Services upper level and middle management changed the policy so that adult clients with severe and persistent mental illness could not be closed unless they were clearly functioning adequately or had moved out of the area. Leadership made this shift from a passive discharge system to the more proactive disease management approach for serving persons with severe and persistent mental illness. Over time directives were given to increase the level of case management, medication subsidies, socialization groups, and long-term supportive care. The utilization management team was developed most recently to help ensure that utilization is analyzed systematically and that there is compliance by the line staff.

The utilization management team devised during the reengineering of the intake and crisis intervention systems has enhanced the utilization management ability of the total agency. In addition to the capability developed at the front end of the system, the utilization management team is developing the ability to 1) identify clients who use a variety and quantity of service, 2) review clients served by the system for more then three years, 3) concurrently review assessments to assure that clinical protocols comply with admissions criteria, 4) review randomly selected open and closed records, and 5) track the speed at which clients are able to initiate treatment. These utilization review strategies evolved over time. In some parts of the system they have yet to be implemented.

While vigilance has increased concerning Behavioral and Mental Health Services' allocation of resources, there remain potential clients at the front door who are not gaining access to the system because dynamic case flow is still inadequate and resource capacity insufficient to meet the need. The no-close policy referred to earlier had to be changed so that clients in the system who are stable at a level of functioning above GAF 45 and are without hospitalization for three years are referred out of the agency. Based on chart review,

116 clients out of 384 were recently selected by the utilization management team and referred to primary care physicians or private practice psychiatrists in order to increase the agency's capacity to serve more seriously ill individuals. This is a work in progress.

ASSESSING THE IMPACT OF SYSTEM REFORM

Many initiatives were conducted over the years. Was there any impact on how the system serves its clients? Over this decade of system reform, waiting time for services to be initiated dropped sharply from 90 days in 1985 to 11.57 days in 1997 (figures include weekends and holidays).

Reduction of hospitalization is a major objective for Behavioral and Mental Health Services. The agency is now the primary gatekeeper for the state psychiatric hospitals. An outcome of lowered hospitalizations reflects the effectiveness of our services. Indicators of the relative level of functioning of the delivery system include state hospital admissions, bed days, and number of successful deflections from the state hospital.

With the assumption of a gatekeeping function for the state hospital, utilization of inpatient care dropped dramatically. Admission rates per 100,000 for both children and adults are displayed in figure 2. In 1988 there were 60 adult admissions per 100,000 population to the state hospital. This declined to 24 adult admissions per 100,000 population in 1997, a 60% decrease in admissions from the DuPage catchment area into the state psychiatric hospital. In FY 1995, DuPage County had 35 adult admissions per 100,000 population, while the regional average was 64 and the state average was 115 admissions per 100,000 population.

In 1989 the admission rate for children and adolescents to the state psychiatric hospital was 21 per 100,000. This was reduced to 2 per 100,000 in 1997, a 91% decrease. The utilization of bed days for children and adolescents declined from 3,014 bed days to 226, or a decrease of 93% (Christian-Michaels, 1995).

Another indicator of success is recidivism as measured by the readmission rate. In the late 1980s the percentage of child clients readmitted after one inpatient stay was more than 11%. A 100% reduction in the readmission of children and adolescents was realized between 1986 and 1997 (see table 2).

A third indicator of success is deflection, that is, the number of children who present at the state psychiatric hospital and are then sent home. There were seventeen deflections in 1989 and zero in 1994. This achievement ensures that children are not exposed to the trauma of an inpatient admission evaluation process that could include seeing adults in acute states of distress.

The last element of assessing the impact of this reform is the support from both internal and external stakeholders. Selling the reform to these stakeholders is perhaps the most difficult task, given the complex web of competing interests. The internal stakeholders included clients, line staff, middle

FIGURE 2   DuPage Public Psychiatric Admits, 1988–1997

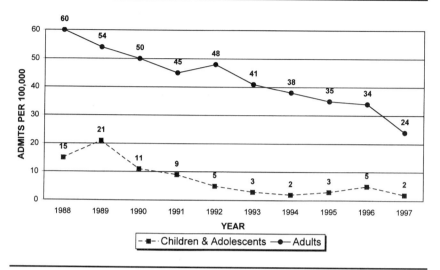

managers, other DuPage County Health Department services, the health department executive director, and the Board of Health. The financial incentives for reform are minimal. Therefore, it was hard to convince the Board of Health, the executive director, and other services of the vital importance of the reform. As the disparities in the missions between public health and community mental health became more evident, Behavioral and Mental Health Services proposed privatizing the agency in order to increase its flexibility and effectiveness in meeting its mission. This has not been realized.

Reorganization of the management structure helped emphasize the importance of meeting the needs of the whole population. The hierarchical structure was replaced with a flat managerial structure in which middle managers met more frequently and had to struggle with client flow problems among themselves. Ultimately, the barrier between upper management and middle management was removed, forming just one management team of seventeen managers. Upper level managers changed their role from consultants to middle managers. Upper level managers were no longer authority figures who approved all decisions. This moved the middle managers into a position of increased autonomy. Middle managers' confidence seems to have increased, while line staff's sense of autonomy has also increased in some units.

It was challenging to convince external stakeholders of the merit of this reform. External stakeholders included the Alliance for the Mentally Ill, the Illinois Department of Human Services Office of Mental Health, other county entities, hospitals, and other community-based service providers. Often the change meant other agencies or community leaders had less influence,

TABLE 2   Average Readmission Rates to Child Public Hospitals

	1986–89	1990–93	1994–97
Average number of readmissions	3	.5	0
Average number of readmissions as percentage of annual admissions	11.12	4.5	0

through personal relationships or political connections, on decisions about services that were allocated by clinical protocols.

A strong relationship was forged with the evolving Alliance for the Mentally Ill (AMI). This relationship started when many AMI members were participants in the psychoeducational series "Facing Mental Illness in the Family." A common understanding about mental illness and the need to band together helped strengthen AMI and acted to increase its membership. AMI began attending all Board of Health meetings and county board meetings, advocating an expansion of services and ultimately privatization.

Several of the majority leaders in the Illinois legislature live in DuPage County. This was used to help leverage support for innovative programs like the crisis unit services, residential services, and case management services.

Strong collaborative relationships were developed with youth service agencies that helped us foster our excellence in serving children and adolescents with severe and persistent mental illness. These cooperative relationships led to joint funding of a twelve-hour day treatment program for youth with conduct disorders.

As the role of gatekeeper to the state hospitals became clearer, a challenge to cooperative relationships emerged. Behavioral and Mental Health Services often refused to recommend admission to the state hospital. Other agencies did not always agree with the proposed alternative services. The assessment staff placed in the position of gatekeeper needed to use their assessment skills, negotiating skills, and public relations skills. Sometimes in successful programs, staff unknowingly become arrogant, too self-assured, and less sensitive to feedback. This continues to be a challenge to be addressed.

SUMMARY

In summary, Behavioral and Mental Health Services has striven to reform our system of care by incubating change and implementing it incrementally. Islands of excellence were created, including a children's hospital gatekeeping and home-based services program, a comprehensive assessment unit, an assertive case management program, and twenty-four-hour access and crisis services. Each of these was a laboratory of change. Innovations also included in-home respite services, extensive use of medication groups and clinics, combined evaluations by the assessor and the psychiatrist, psychoeducational programs, and a treatment package manual that depicts arrays of service with multiple levels of care. The innovations were not only mirrored internally but were also modeled by other community mental health agencies across Illinois and in other states.

Innovation was constrained by being part of a much larger public bureaucracy. This position contributed to the agency's inability to use increased revenues to expand existing program capacity. Given the political need to lower local real estate taxes, few avenues for increasing program capacity remain. In spite of being part of a large, static bureaucracy, excellence was achieved in many arenas. Though resources to serve this most at-risk population were very scarce, fewer and fewer clients depended on the state psychiatric hospitals. With changes to welfare, managed Medicaid, managed Medicare, and, potentially, block grants, the test is whether these managed care applications will continue to differentiate who needs what care and at what level. Such care must be delivered quickly in a manner that helps the clients obtain high-quality services and where outcome indicators assess the effectiveness of treatment, driving further system reform.

REFERENCES

American Psychiatric Association. (1994). *Diagnostic and statistical manual of mental disorders (4th ed.)*. Washington, DC: Author.

Christian-Michaels, S. (1995). Psychiatric emergencies and family preservation: Partnership in an array of community-based services. In L. Combrink-Graham (Ed.), *Children in families at risk: Maintaining the connections*. New York: Guilford.

DuPage County Health Department. (1997). A treatment package manual. Unpublished internet document, DuPage County Health Department, Behavioral and Mental Health Services.

Endicott, J., Spritzer, R. L., Fleiss, J., & Coehn, J. (1976). The Global Assessment Scale: A procedure for measuring overall severity of psychiatric disturbance. *Archives of General Psychiatry, 33,* 766–771.

Hoge, M. A., Davidson, L., Griffith, E. E., Sledge, W. H., & Howenstine, R. A. (1994). Defining managed care in public-sector psychiatry. *Hospital and Community Psychiatry, 45*(11), 1085–1089.

Shaffer, D., Gould, M. S., Brasic, J., et. al. (1983). A Children's Global Assessment Scale (CGAS). *Archives of General Psychiatry, 40,* 1228–1231.

Torrey, E. F., & Wolfe, S. M. (1990). *Care of the seriously mentally ill: A rating of state programs*. Washington, DC: Public Citizen Health Research Group.

PART THREE

The Changing Therapeutic Relationship

This final part of the book contains a single chapter and an epilogue. The chapter is a conceptual analysis of the impact of managed care on the therapeutic relationship. Crotty places the therapeutic, human service relationship within a larger societal context. He looks at the influence that the changing, temporizing economy has on interpersonal interaction in social work treatment. Crotty sees a fundamental change in interpersonal interactions within the larger society mirrored in the therapeutic process.

CHAPTER 10

Relationships, Encounters and the Corporate Culture in Managed Mental Health Care

Patrick Crotty

Assistant Professor, School of Social Work,
Loyola University Chicago

There is growing evidence that many mental health professionals are becoming dissatisfied with managed care and its restrictive demands. Concerns are expressed about such matters as short hospital stays, fewer and briefer psychotherapy sessions, loss of professional autonomy, reduced incomes, contracts that "gag" professionals, and a variety of other issues. I suggest that these concerns are merely a symptom of a paradigm shift and focusing on them may obscure the larger picture, namely, that as the provision of mental health services becomes a business enterprise it will inevitably take on the characteristics of such an enterprise. This chapter will speak to the current dehumanizing of these very personal interactions and to the movement toward the nontherapeutic encounter. It will focus on the shift in health care to a business enterprise and will discuss how the customary professional relationship in mental health care is moving toward a new characterization of the provider—customer transaction, that is, the service encounter.

RELATIONSHIPS AND ENCOUNTERS

In her study of divergent philosophies of social interaction Gutek (1995) notes the kinds of changes currently taking place in customer-provider relationships. She distinguishes bureaucratic encounters, where people remain strangers to each other, from personal relationships, where people come to know one another as individuals.

A relationship, in Gutek's terms, implies frequent, enduring, and often lengthy interactions. An attachment is formed and trust is developed, and there is an element of mutual dependency. Both parties are committed to the relationship and are concerned for each other. They also develop shared knowledge that is specific and nontransferable. So, for example, a psychotherapist comes to know the particular problems, needs, interests, and concerns of the client, which enhances over time, the efficiency and effectiveness of their relationship. This learning process has to be replicated with each new client. Relationships are labor intensive. Relationships can also be a source of mutual satisfaction and enjoyment, and some status may even accrue to the participants, as well as a sense of ownership, so that people speak of *my* client or *my* doctor or *my* therapist.

The encounter has no continuity or permanence of interaction, unlike the relationship, which rests on a history of shared interaction. Nor does it enable or encourage the knowledge of the other's expectations or needs that comes with a relationship, nor does it allow wide variation in the pattern of responses to account for customer differences. In the encounter providers (and customers) are interchangeable. Their unique qualities are irrelevant to their jobs.

In the service industry the encounter is the primary means by which service resources are exchanged between provider and customer. It calls for the presence of both parties, and both share in the transaction. No prior relationship is required, and task-related information dominates the exchange. It is, as Czepiel, Solomon, Surprenant, and Gutman note, "a socially sanctioned relationship between strangers" (1985, p. 5). Service encounters are vitally important to conducting business and to the whole notion of quality assurance, especially because they are perceived by the customer as a large part of the product offered (Czepiel et al., 1985; Shostack, 1985; Bowen, & Pearson, 1992).

It is not always necessary to have a relationship with the provider of services. If we are making a business transaction, an encounter may be preferred. We may simply want to get the job done as quickly and as efficiently as possible. Hence the advantage of the ATM. It may be neither necessary nor wise to spend three or four dollars to talk to a bank teller. Skopec (1996) suggest that the provision of counseling to bank customers is being replaced by "faceless interactions" and that "relationships are being sacrificed in favor of transactions." Even financial institutions, however, are becoming aware of problems arising from excessive dependence on encounters, particularly in situations where it may be important to develop a more personal relationship with a client.

While both relationships and encounters may serve us well, depending on the context, I believe that the distinction raises serious questions, given the nature of the work that mental health professionals do. The relationship between the therapist and the client is seen as pivotal. It is generally accepted that no real change can be effected until the relationship has been established. With the increasing emphasis of managed care organizations on efficiency and productivity, professional relationships in mental health care appear to be moving in the direction of service encounters, and the human interaction that has always been accepted as integral to that relationship is being degraded.

FACTORS FAVORING THE ENCOUNTER MODE

Professional Practice Factors

A number of factors may be seen as contributing to this deterioration of the professional relationship in managed health care. From the perspective of professional practice, three such factors may be noted: the emergence of brief treatment, the separation of payment from service, and the growing workload.

Brief treatment is rapidly emerging as the psychotherapeutic treatment of choice in managed health care. However plausible the reasons for reducing the number and length of therapy hours (and most of the reasons will fall under the rubric of cost containment or efficiency), this change can be expected to offer severely reduced opportunities for shared interaction. It is unlikely that in such situations time will be allowed for the development of understanding and trust and for the kind of commitment normally associated with a relationship.

The separation of payment from the provision of service, as in the case of non–fee-for-service arrangements, further weakens the link between service provider and client. When clients do not personally pay the fee, they are likely to value the service less and to invest less in the treatment process. Moreover, when people pay money to join a health plan such as a health maintenance organization, the organization receives payment whether or not a client receives any particular service. More clients may merely mean more work for the same pay. As Gutek (1995) observes, "The wishes or needs of the customer are likely to get less attention when payment is authorized by and comes from a source other than the customer, than when the customer either authorizes payment or pays directly" (p. 77).

The ability to establish a relationship may also be related to the size of the workload. A small number of customers allows the development of more personal relationships, while serving a large number will likely call for the encounter mode. Seventy-five percent of insured workers are now in managed care plans, compared with 50% in 1994, an increase of 25% in less than three years ("HMOs Cover," 1997). Individual managed care organizations have grown in size while decreasing in number as the market has consolidated through acquisitions and mergers. In 1993, the seventeen largest managed behavioral health care carve-out companies together covered some 80 million lives (Trabin & Freeman, 1995). Inevitably managed care providers will have larger practices, so that many interactions will be encounters because the parties will have no opportunities to build relationships and indeed may be unsure if they will ever meet again. And we may be moving toward a situation where clinicians will become functionally equivalent, so that the therapist you see today may not be the one you see tomorrow because all are doing the same thing and following the same service protocols.

Functional equivalence or substitutability may be more likely to affect poor clients, who are unable to purchase "gold card" health care options that would entitle them to more extended services. As Gutek (1995) points out, "The premium often paid for relationship interactions means that many poor people are unable to afford anything but an encounter option" (p. 249). Also, the services that low-income people seek when they apply for various benefits—public aid, food stamps, energy assistance, and so forth—are generally offered only in the encounter mode. Governments and other organizations believe this mode to be the most efficient and therefore the least expensive. The disadvantaged clients are given no choice in the matter. To the extent that managed care forces people into encounters rather than relationships, therapists and other social service providers become another faceless bureaucracy to the marginalized in our society—more so, as managed care is applied to public sector programs.

Industrial and Bureaucratic Factors

Significant external forces appear to be transforming the relationship into the encounter mode. The importation of industrial and bureaucratic models into the fields of health, mental health, and social services are contributing to this major change. Driven largely by cost containment, such modes strongly emphasize efficiency and rationality along with increased technological monitoring. The technological goal is to raise the number of patients or clients while simultaneously cutting costs. It requires the standardization of treatment practices, clients, and service providers in order to increase the efficiency of production (Fisher & Karger, 1997). Consistency and dependability are expected. Variability in work processes becomes less acceptable. These processes are designed to accommodate the strengths of a cost-effective technology and are restructuring the relationship between customer and client (Fabricant & Burghardt, 1992). Mental health professionals who place a high value on human interaction now find themselves culturally and philosophically at odds with models that tend to replace professional relationships with service encounters or transactions.

Ritzer (1993) argues that the principles of the fast food industry are beginning to take hold in many areas of American society, including education and health care. He finds the antecedents of this "McDonaldization" in Weber's concept of bureaucracy, Taylor's principles of scientific management, and Ford's invention of the assembly line. In Max Weber's concept of formal rationality, tried and tested means to a given end are "institutionalized in rules, regulations and structures" (Ritzer, 1993, p. 19). So, whether in the field of health or fast food, a streamlined process is developed in which employees follow clearly defined rules that, while limiting provider and consumer choices, tend nevertheless to maximize efficiency.

Even though management in the nineties has moved well beyond the principles enunciated by Frederick W. Taylor, it is Ritzer's contention that Taylor's ideas continue to shape the way work is now performed in the fast food industry and in other industries such as health care. Taylor expounded the notion that "every single act of every workman can be reduced to a science" (Taylor, 1947, p. 64) so that any piece of work can be broken down into a series of prescribed tasks that can therefore be predicted and controlled. So, for example, a counseling agency may focus on the various processes involved in getting a client into treatment—the initial telephone call, the waiting period, the initial clinical interview, the business office interview, and so on.

Finally, the assembly line as developed by Henry Ford and others, with its efficient but dehumanizing aspects, again had the effect of breaking work down into its simplest components, ensuring maximum control with minimum product variability. First widely used in the manufacturing industry, this type of work routinization later came to be applied to clerical work as it grew in importance. With the rapid expansion of the service sector, job standardization has now expanded into the area of interactive service work, or jobs that require workers to have face-to-face relationships with clients.

The appeal of work routinization or standardization and the application of scientific management and related principles lies in their promise of efficiency, calculability, predictability, and control (Ritzer, 1993). While primarily thought of in relation to the fast food industry and other work domains, I believe that these four factors have particular relevance to our understanding of some of the revolutionary changes currently taking place in the field of managed health care.

Efficiency. "Efficiency" means choosing the quickest and cheapest means to an end. In managed managed health care it means obtaining the best possible outcomes at the least cost while maintaining quality care. In order to achieve this end it becomes necessary to develop a technology that can be operationalized in specific rules and regulations that service providers can be required to follow: find out what really works and then have everybody do the same thing. This is clearly a difficult task in the complex area of managed health care. In psychotherapy, for example, it is the relationship that is seen as the vehicle for change, and the obvious difficulties involved in attempting to standardize relationships create serious efficiency problems.

Leidner (1993) addresses this issue and notes that all interactive service work will have some noninteractive component that may be comparatively easy to standardize. Even psychotherapy involves "off-stage" interactive tasks such as completing forms. However, when the interaction moves beyond these more easily formalized processes, any effort to routinize must in some way involve the therapists themselves.

Hochschild (1983) notes "the rise of the corporate use of guile and the organized training of feelings to sustain it" (p. 43). In the interests of efficiency therapists are encouraged to change their ways of thinking and to adapt to changing circumstances in their field. Mental health organization administrators are urged to get the necessary structures and systems in place so as to create an effective and efficient organization capable of competing in the current climate. Meanwhile, therapists struggle to maintain their own definitions of their clients' health and well-being in the context of their own professional values, aspirations, and ethical standards (Cornelius, 1994).

In time, these demands for efficiency must begin to affect the way therapists represent themselves to their clients. Managed care organizations' attempts to routinize the professional relationship can become a way of seeking to rationalize therapists' self-presentation, as well as their feelings and behaviors. For example, while good clinical guidelines can be helpful to therapist and client, they may also lead to the development of "pseudorelationships" (Gutek, 1995), in which use of methods and techniques developed by others may bring about an attempt to personalize routines and simulate authenticity—a behavior altogether out of place in a client-therapist relationship.

With the erosion of professional autonomy therapists may begin to question their authenticity and their use of self in the therapeutic situation. The gradual intrusion of the market may critically affect how they define themselves, and as representatives of the company with which they or their agency have a contract, they may find themselves becoming agents of managed social control. Indeed, with heightened external expectations, being an agent of the company may be more important than the kind of therapeutic authenticity or spontaneity that has been a key characteristic of the psychotherapeutic relationship.

Personal or organizational ideologies may also prove to be obstacles to change and to achieving the desired level of efficiency. Different social service agencies, as well as individual practitioners, will have somewhat different theoretical positions, as they relate to their clients. And since practice ideologies are often derived from these theoretical and moral positions, whether of the organization or of the individual or both, practice orientations will likely vary according to these ideologies and frustrate corporate attempts at organizational efficiency (Hasenfeld, 1974).

Finally, the very nature of the social service organization or the character of the therapeutic practice may raise barriers to bureaucratic efficiency. "Machine bureaucracy" that is generated to create efficiency is likely to be vertically structured with all of the most important decisions made at the top. "Professional bureaucracy," on the other hand, tends to be flatter, more decentralized, with the individual having considerably more autonomy. Attempts, therefore, to standardize professional behaviors in the interests of efficiency, whether by means of policies, monitoring, or protocols, will likely meet considerable resistance and disturb the professional-client relationship (Bolman & Deal, 1991). The "presence" of third- or even fourth-party players in the therapeutic situation must inevitably affect the therapeutic interaction, given the constant monitoring, the numerous demands, the procedural expectations, as well as the ethical, moral, and occupational conflicts generated by this kind of intrusive oversight.

Calculability.   Things get done more quickly and efficiently when measurement or "calculability" is involved. Even in the best of circumstances quantity may take the place of quality; volume of business may take precedence over care. Quantification often becomes an important item on the cost reduction and containment agenda. It includes setting time limits for patient office visits, limiting the number of times a psychotherapy client may be seen, and maximizing the number of patients or clients who may be seen. Quantification also includes the assessment of effectiveness or impact using outcome measures and the measurement of customer satisfaction using client surveys.

Good outcome measures have consistently eluded the providers of managed health care. The push for such measures by managed care companies may serve the very useful purpose of forcing providers to pay attention to and examine the effectiveness of their work. Unfortunately, measures of outcome are sometimes used by managed care organizations more with a view to the marketing of their product than with any concern about employing a valid and reliable instrument to demonstrate the effectiveness of an intervention.

Measures of client or customer satisfaction have been underutilized by mental health practitioners. This may be due to the traditional bias of researchers against client self-report or to the belief of clinicians that clients are unable to gauge the level of their own dysfunction. Even though they may sometimes elicit socially desirable responses, satisfaction surveys do have a useful function in allowing clients to respond to and have some input into the therapeutic process.

Regardless of the measure, whether it is of outcome or satisfaction, there are obvious cognitive and emotional aspects to the professional relationship that are highly intangible and difficult to formalize. Siehl et al. (1992) note two specific issues in the service encounter affecting both the service provider and the customer that are obstacles to calculability.

First, in the case of highly intangible services where the product is not separable from the person providing it, such as psychotherapy, the client becomes a major source of "input uncertainty" for the provider. The latter needs to process the information received from the customer, information being the primary raw material that he has to work with. For the worker in a fast food service or the clerk in a retail store, this does not normally present a problem. They are dealing with a very tangible product. However, it becomes a serious issue for the provider of mental health services, and because of the possible negative consequences of this kind of uncertainty for efficiency and profitability in the field of managed care, management will seek to develop procedural mechanisms to ensure the kind of input specificity that makes outcome measurement possible.

Second, from the point of view of the client or the customer, the highly intangible and ambiguous nature of such services makes it difficult to make the kind of judgment necessary to evaluate the services, even after they have been received. Furthermore, the cognitive and emotional aspects of the process will affect clients' responses to the service; they may either give the service a high rating based on their own investment of time and effort in the process or they may have a negative response because of the perceived painfulness of the process. Either way their evaluation of the services received will be of questionable validity.

Predictability. With increased standardization of the treatment process "predictability" becomes more possible. Predictability implies the ability to generate the same product across time and location. The Big Mac you purchase in Baltimore today will be identical with the one served to you in San Francisco tomorrow. A specific mental health problem will be treated in the same way and have the same outcome regardless of where or when the therapy is carried out.

Traditionally, the practice of behavioral health care has been short on predictability. Clinicians have tended to pride themselves on their eclecticism. Although a number of studies in recent years suggest that the overall effects of psychotherapy have been positive, research has determined only a limited number of situations in which a specific treatment procedure is effective for a particular problem, and there is little evidence to suggest that any one form of therapy is better than any other (Austad, 1996).

Social workers tend to accept the concept of "practice wisdom" more than empirically based knowledge. Clinicians for the most part have not experienced organizational or professional association constraints that might have made their approaches to treatment more predictable. The field has been relatively free of externally mandated treatment guidelines or demands for evidence of success, resulting in a considerable lack of accountability (Wylie, 1994).

With more emphasis on profitability there is likely to be a growing expectation of predictability. Pressure to contain costs will demand a greater degree of formalization and more decisions will rest with bureaucracies—third-party payers and state and federal governments—to ensure a greater level of conformity. This process of rationalization may well mean that providers will have less control over their work and be likely to experience greater job dissatisfaction and alienation.

It may also lead to some degree of deprofessionalization of psychotherapy as a result of a diminution of the power and control that practitioners have over their work. There is an autonomy threshold below which one may cease to be a professional. The growing demand for predictability is also likely to affect clients. Rules and guidelines that call for a high level of treatment conformity must ultimately affect, and inevitably diminish, the personal professional relationship.

Control.   The fourth factor is control, particularly in the areas of utilization and variability. "Utilization" relates to the amount of services used by clients. Managed care organizations seek to control utilization of services by various review procedures. These may be carried out prospectively to demonstrate the necessity of or to authorize treatment, concurrently to monitor ongoing treatment, or retrospectively to determine treatment outcomes (Corcoran & Vandiver, 1996). Cornelius (1994) suggests that in order to control utilization every behavioral health service offered is under the monitoring eye of a case manager. Service utilization needs to be controlled since managed care succeeds only to the extent that careful surveillance of a provider's practice is carried out. This is achieved by having every case structured according to the protocols of the managed care company. Case management becomes a form of surveillance to encourage or enforce compliance. The service provider, by entering into the contract, "becomes an agent of managed care and agrees to serve the public within the corporate guidelines and not necessarily according to the assessed needs of the client" (Cornelius, 1994, p. 51).

It is also arguable that there are considerably more structural and interactional constraints on therapists in managed care than in traditional indemnity health plans. Managed care organizations seek to build information databases on therapists' practice patterns using utilization reviews, outcome studies, and consumer satisfaction surveys. Surveillance therefore seems to be much more intrusive. The therapist is constantly being judged on his or her compliance through frequent reports and repeated contacts with case managers.

The therapist has to balance possibly conflicting interests—the clinician's professional assessment, the needs of the client, and the expectations of the managed care organization. Advocacy tends to become narrowly defined in terms of making a case for additional sessions for the client rather than in the much broader context of structural intervention or change. Failure to obtain additional sessions when the therapist deems this to be clinically appropriate can raise major ethical and moral issues. There is strong pressure, especially in staff model health maintenance organizations, "to wring the most mental health product out of every allotted clinical hour" (Wylie, 1994, p. 25).

Minimizing and controlling "variability" are at the heart of the success of the managed health care enterprise. Variability goes hand in hand with cost. The greater the variability the greater the cost, whether it relates to the amount of meat in a hamburger or to the kinds of surgical procedures used in a specific operation or to the intervention used in treating a particular psychological problem.

Variability or process variation constitutes a major threat to the product or service produced by that process (Bartlett, 1994). Clinical processes such as psychotherapy often have a wide degree of variability or flexibility. Normal variations are to be expected and are acceptable as long as they fall within some defined limits. It is wide fluctuations that are cause for concern to the health care industry. Bartlett (1994) notes that these fluctuations are often associated with ill-defined, poorly understood, and badly managed processes and suggests that in the delivery of mental health and substance abuse services we are in fact trying to manage processes for which no standards exist and that standards are needed to detect and control unacceptable variation.

Related to this is the issue of clinical standards, protocols, or "best practices" that service providers find to be problematic as externally imposed controls. One can hardly quarrel with clinical guidelines that are based not merely on the consensus of clinicians (it is possible that they could all be wrong) but also on sound research. Such standards may have an important function in protecting clients by using state-of-the-art treatment approaches and by informing the judgment of case managers as they review cases (Bartlett, 1994, p. 160). Yet there is some concern about the use of such guidelines to the extent that they are another piece of the routinization of behavioral health care. They may lead to a "cookbook" approach to the practice of psychotherapy and stifle innovative clinical practice.

A further issue is the "one size fits all" approach that can be a temptation in managed care organizations. For example, short-term psychotherapy cannot be the standard for everyone regardless of problem severity or clinical diagnosis. There may well be a need for clinically appropriate long-term psychotherapy, and clients may be seen to deserve treatment that is tailored to their clinical needs. This conflict between the need for managed care companies to ration health care and use prescriptive guidelines for cost containment purposes and the need for clinicians to provide the kind of care for which the assessment and diagnosis calls is a source of ethical dilemmas for many practitioners.

A question can also be raised as to how serious the managed care industry is in the use of such best practices. There may well be a mixed message. While apparently interested in sound practice guidelines, in proper provider credentials, and in philosophy of treatment, managed care organizations may, at the same time, give providers the impression that once the contract is signed the really important thing is to have the treatment carried out as expeditiously as possible, with little concern for the quality of the relationship.

Treatment protocols have often been company secrets. Recently, some managed care companies have made them available or published them. It is likely that they have made their criteria public in response to the anger of practitioners since secret criteria represent a "stacked deck" in the patient review process. To date, however, there appears to be little evidence that making review guidelines available will lead to clinical manipulation on the part of practitioners, to arbitrary restriction of reimbursement on the part of payers, or to exploitation by attorneys or litigious patients initiating malpractice proceedings (McIntyre, 1994).

Given these various ways in which managed care seeks to standardize and control mental health care using numerous demands and procedural expectations, and given the ethical, moral, and occupational conflicts generated in service providers in various disciplines, it is inevitable that the professional therapist-client relationship will be in some way affected.

ETHICS AND ENCOUNTERS

Ethical concerns will invariably arise when the culture of the marketplace clashes with that of the mental health service provider. One might argue that a market philosophy, by its very nature, conflicts with the beneficent-oriented value system of a human service provider or organization. The fiduciary duty to the client may conflict with the contractual obligation to the service purchaser when, as they often are, they are not one and the same. There should be concern about the shift of financial control to a nonclinical, corporate entity and the extent to which the values of the corporate world may undermine the best interests of the client (Corcoran & Vandiver, 1996).

Ethical issues may be quite challenging within the changing context of the therapeutic relationship. Mention has already been made of the erosion of the practitioner's autonomy and the struggle to maintain authenticity in the face of externally imposed guidelines and mandates. As third and fourth parties attain more influence in the clinical decision-making process, the therapist may feel that his or her ethical standards and values are compromised and the fiduciary duty to the client undermined. Confidentiality may be strained by pervasive management surveillance. Growing dependence on short-term treatment and overzealous cost cutting may create an ever present danger of client abandonment, especially for those whose problems are severe.

The ethical concerns, however, go beyond these to more fundamental issues—priority setting and rationing. Prioritization of service provision due to scarcity of resources is a fact of life. Who receives care, what kind of care, and for how long is no less an ethical dilemma for the fee-for-service practitioner than it is for a practitioner in an organization working under a capitated contract. Decisions about the provision and intensity of care are made routinely, whether on the basis of income or personal preference or government funding or happenstance. Inevitably, clinicians are participating in a rationing process that is no less real for being invisible.

Mental health agencies frequently find themselves having to assist large numbers of clients with resources that are inadequate—usually in the form of inadequate numbers of direct service providers who may have neither the time nor the expertise to provide optimal interventions. There may be a clear awareness that a more intensive psychotherapeutic approach might yield more permanent results and even bring about a significant reduction, over the long term, in financial as well as social costs. However, long-term therapy may be an unaffordable luxury. Forced into client interactions that tend to be in the encounter mode, agencies may have to adopt modes of intervention that are likely to have a population rather than an individualized focus, emphasizing community care rather than more traditional relationship therapy. Oftentimes managed care merely institutionalizes this treatment approach. And the more sophisticated forms of psychotherapy that individuals with greater financial resources may be able to purchase will not normally be made available to mental health agency clients.

Clinical social workers and other therapists may see such encounter-type treatment as second rate. They may even feel that clients are being cheated and ought in fact be able to receive more in-depth and intensive forms of treatment if this is what they need or even seek. However, to expect such care for the large numbers of people of all ages with mental health problems serious enough to call for professional assistance is to assume the availability of many competent clinicians who can demonstrate positive outcomes through their interventions.

To routinize in-depth, intensive treatment formats is also to assume the availability of extraordinary levels of funding. It is unrealistic to suppose that funding will be available for expensive forms of treatment that may well be only marginally more effective. This is not to say that population-focused or community care approaches are inexpensive. Chronicity and recidivism, and their concomitant costs, are not about to go away. Nevertheless, the emphasis on and funding for case management, medication management, and various other forms of social care and prevention services may continue to offer the best hope for the majority of those with serious mental illness (Quinlivan et al., 1995). The extent to which managed care will support this approach is dubious. Unfortunately, it remains one of the ironies and injustices of this issue that high administrative costs and excessive profit making are rarely called into question.

What, then, of the issue of social and economic justice for recipients of mental health care? What does it mean to be a "just and caring society" at a time when resources are limited and health needs virtually unlimited? Fleck (1994) is of the opinion that the provision of care ought not to be determined on the basis of an invisible agenda but rather that priorities should be determined on the basis of a democratic ranking process. A recent American Medical Association document suggests that practitioners may need to consider individual claims in the light of the competing demands of other patients to available resources (American Medical Association, 1995). This perspective seems to incorporate economic realities and issues of social justice.

On what basis, then, do we decide who gets care, or more specifically, who gets care beyond an encounter mode? Given the many levels of need and problem severity, and the scarcity of resources, how are priorities to be determined? Darr (1987) offers four ethical principles for health service management that have relevance in this context. They are the principles of autonomy, beneficence, nonmaleficence, and justice. Autonomy calls for respect for the right of individual choice. Individuals are the final authority for their own health care decisions. They should have the freedom to select their service providers, and participate in decisions regarding their own health. Beneficence means that the providers of health or mental health services will act in the best interest of clients and advocate on their behalf. It articulates the fiduciary responsibility to clients who depend on the provider and must trust that their interests will be served. Nonmaleficence is a restating of the moral principle that no harm be done to the client. No risk should be taken unless the potential results justify it (Vanstone, 1995). Justice, and more specifically distributive justice, calls for giving to each according to his or her need and includes the concept of fairness in the allocation of resources. Depending on the particular circumstances or ethical issue these principles may be weighed or ordered differently. Nevertheless, they can provide a useful guide for discussing ethical dilemmas associated with priority setting.

Austed (1996), writing from the "societal ethic" perspective, notes that the best interests of the individual may not always serve the common good and that we ought to be guided by justice rather than by autonomy. She perceives the principles of autonomy and beneficence as individually oriented and having to do more with individual than collective rights. She also believes that many of the managed care issues about which therapists are concerned are essentially issues of individual rights—confidentiality, client abandonment, utilization review, precertification, and so forth. This is not to diminish the importance of these concerns but rather to ensure that they are perceived in a broader societal context.

Within the context of the therapeutic relationship, the question as to who gets what level of care can be reframed: to what extent does the caring relationship need to be modified in the interests of justice? Naturally those with personal financial resources will purchase the type of therapeutic relationship they desire. While individuals may have a right to basic mental health care, nobody has an absolute right either to unlimited access to that care or to unlimited care. To allow such rights would inevitably infringe on the rights of others who may have an equal or even greater claim to such resources. Whether it is an insurance plan, a health maintenance organization, or governmental contracted services, overutilization by some will deplete the resources that are available to others.

The encounter, therefore, may be seen as a modification of the relationship and, in the collective interest, will be called for in certain circumstances. Decisions will need to take into account the severity and duration of the problem, the demonstrated effectiveness of the intervention, and the cost of the intervention. Treatments that are marginally effective are unlikely to benefit anyone, regardless of cost or problem severity. The more difficult decisions will center on effective but expensive interventions for high-severity problems. Justice is not served by offering expensive, long-term relationships to those with relatively minor disorders or by the inappropriate use of encounters for those with severe impairments. Justice is rather served by the appropriate use of encounters and relationships based on clearly stated, predetermined priorities.

Ultimately, then, it comes down to being able to maintain a balance among individualistic and collective rights and obligations. The building and maintenance of relationships has to be tempered by an awareness of economic realities. A beneficence that is concerned only with the best interests of the individual and an expectation of unlimited practitioner-client autonomy ignores the wider claims of distributive justice. Ethical practice will mean a constant struggle between these elements—limiting but not excluding client choice and serving and promoting the best interests of the individual without ignoring the claims of the many.

POSITIVE ASPECTS OF ENCOUNTERS

While professionals may well lament the apparent passing of the therapeutic relationship, from the customer's point of view there may be some real advantages to having predictable, efficient, and measurable products. In almost every aspect of their lives customers have become aware of these advantages, whether it be in relation to fast food, convenience stores, rapid transit, ATMs, or walk-in emergency health care centers. Medical patients may well prefer to go to a storefront "intermediate health care center" where they do not need an appointment and will be likely to get prompt and efficient service, rather than to a private physician, even though they will not get the kind of personal attention and ongoing relationship that the latter might provide. There are indications that clients appear to be generally satisfied with managed health care services (Braus, 1994), suggesting that people may feel they are receiving good health care at an affordable price in managed care plans and that they may even be willing to sacrifice choice for this.

In mental health care, clients are more likely to be smart shoppers than they were a decade ago. In seeking counseling or psychotherapy for themselves or their families, they are more likely to ask such questions as "How long will it take?" "How much will it cost" or "What exactly will you do for me?" These can be difficult questions for psychotherapists with a psychodynamic orientation who in the early stages of treatment may be unable to make a reliable judgment about length of treatment and consequently about the overall cost to the client. It is indeed arguable that long-term psychotherapy is no longer a marketable commodity, not only from the perspective of the managed care organization, which perceives it not to be cost effective, but even from the point of view of the client, who accustomed to efficiently organized systems may not find the time, money, or inclination to become involved in this type of treatment.

Many see these new and more efficient systems in a positive light, perceiving them as offering greater availability of goods and services, shorter waiting lines, convenient hours, fast service, and even the likelihood of more equitable treatment, regardless of their race, social class, or gender (Ritzer, 1993). Leidner (1993) notes the practical benefits of routinization both to service workers and recipients and suggests that it can help workers to do their jobs better, boost their confidence, and limit the demands that customers place on them. Customers or clients may obtain more reliable, faster, and less expensive service while being protected from incompetence and negative interactions.

CONCLUSION

As practitioners of psychotherapy and mental health agencies seek to make the changes they deem necessary to survive in an era of managed care, there may be little time to think about important by-products of these changes, especially those that are not immediately obvious, such as those subtle but significant changes in the provider-client relationship. Nevertheless, these subtle shifts are of considerable import for helping professionals since they may affect the whole character of their work. Practitioners need to be acutely aware of the variety of changes taking place in their world and especially of the impact of economic and sociological developments on what they do.

The ever changing nature of the managed mental health care environment makes prediction difficult. However, professional survival may depend on having the ability to discern future trends and directions. Some see little future for long-term psychotherapy as we now know it, even perceiving it to be unethical since the extended use of a service by one person, assuming a limited pool of scarce resources, may mean that another person is deprived of care (Austad, 1996). Others are of the opinion that it is possible to continue to provide good, clinical psychotherapeutic services in the business environment of managed care while maintaining one's professional values and integrity (Harris, 1996). And there are those who see "intermittent" therapy as the therapy of the future, wherein clients may return many times for brief therapy over the course of their lives. In this way the relationship may persist in the absence of traditional long-term treatment (Austad, 1996; Cummings, 1996; Hoyt, 1996).

Ultimately, however, forces beyond the control of professionals may define the future. Gutek (1995) suggests a number of factors that are likely to facilitate the growth of encounters. Three of these factors will be briefly considered here as most likely to affect the provision of mental health care as we move into a new century.

The first is of particular interest and has already been alluded to; it has to do with the perception and experience of the young. Customers growing up in the changing world of the health maintenance organization, solution-focused therapy, the drive-in bank, the "doc in the box" medical center, the fast food restaurant, and the Jiffy Lube may neither have nor desire the kind of long-term relationships that their parents enjoyed with doctors, lawyers, motor mechanics, bankers, or therapists. Many of them have worked in encounter-type jobs, made their purchases, eaten their meals, and obtained their health care in encounter situations. Their lifestyles and their stretched incomes may not permit the luxury of anything more.

Second is the growing practice of professionals' and experts' withdrawing from direct work with customers or clients. These professionals tend to delegate much of their direct service roles to others, whether nurses in hospitals, teaching assistants in colleges or universities, physician assistants or nurses in health maintenance organizations, or case managers in social service agencies. As these newer and less costly occupations continue to substitute for traditional professions, customers may find themselves more satisfied with the encounters offered by these alternative providers, "especially if encounters are less expensive and encounter providers are more courteous, pleasant, and cheerful in dispensing service" (Gutek, 1995, p. 266).

Finally, some market and demographic trends deserve notice. The ongoing development of management as a field independent of any particular area of expertise is begetting a breed of "general purpose managers" for whom the encounter is likely to be the major modus operandi. Divorced from any particular specialty their style is unlikely to be one that calls for the development of relationships with clients or customers.

The continuing growth of urban areas and declining sense of community will tend to preclude the kind of professional and business relationships that one might observe in small towns or rural areas. When the population is sparse and time is not such a highly valued commodity, relationships are more likely to flourish. And if we also take into account present-day geographical mobility and the increasing demands on the time of two-income families, the future of relationship development with mental health professionals may seem doubtful.

As these trends continue, will we witness an increasing erosion of professional relationships as we now know them? As young people age, will they seek more than mere transactions with professionals and other service providers? And even if they do, will anything more than an encounter be available to them unless they have the income and the time to afford it? These are open questions. Nevertheless, they do suggest that however much mental health care professionals may lament the passing of the therapeutic relationship, what happens in the future may not be entirely up to them.

REFERENCES

American Medical Association. (1995). Ethical issues in managed care. *Journal of the American Medical Association, 273*(4), 330–335.

Austad, C. S. (1996). *Is long-term psychotherapy unethical? Toward a social ethic in an era of managed care.* San Francisco: Jossey-Bass.

Bartlett, J. (1994). Practice guidelines: The managed care view. In R. K. Schreter, S. S. Sharfstein, & C. A. Schreter (Eds.), *Allies and adversaries: The impact of managed care on mental health services* (pp. 153–162). Washington, DC: American Psychiatric Press.

Bolman, L. G., & Deal, T. E. (1991). *Reframing organizations: Artistry, choice, and leadership.* San Francisco: Jossey-Bass.

Braus, P. (1994). HMOs get high marks from their members. *American Demographics, 16*(2), 17–18.

Cornelius, D. S. (1994). Managed care and social work: Constructing a context and a response. *Social Work in Health Care, 20*(1), 47–63.

Corcoran, K., & Vandiver, V. (1996). *Manuevering the maze of managed care: Skills for mental health practitioners.* New York: Free Press.

Cummings, N. A. (1996). The impact of managed care on employment and professional training. A primer for survival. In N. A. Cummings, M. S. Pallak, & J. L. Cummings (Eds.), *Surviving the demise of solo practice: Mental health practitioners prospering in the era of managed care* (pp. 11–26). Madison, WI: Psychosocial Press.

Czepiel, J. A., Solomon, M. R., Surprenant, C. F., & Gutman, E. G. (1985). Service encounters: An overview: In J. A. Czepiel, M. R. Solomon, & C. F. Surprenant (Eds.), *The service encounter: Managing employee/customer interaction in service businesses* (pp. 3–16). Lexington, MA: Lexington.

Darr, K. (1987). *Ethics in health services management* (2nd ed.). Baltimore: Health Professions Press.

Fabricant, M., & Burghardt, S. (1992). *The welfare state crisis and the transformation of social service work.* Armonk, NY: Sharpe.

Fisher, R., & Karger, H. J. (1997). *Social work and community in a private world: Getting out in public.* White Plains, NY: Longman.

Fleck, L. (1994). Just caring: Oregon, health care rationing, and informed democratic deliberation. *Journal of Medicine and Philosophy, 19,* 367–388.

Gutek, B. A. (1995). *The dynamics of service: Reflections on the changing nature of customer/provider interactions.* San Francisco: Jossey-Bass.

Harris. S. O. (1996). The practitioner as clinician: The business of practice. In N. A. Cummings, M. S. Pallak, & J. L. Cummings (Eds.), *Surviving the demise of solo practice: Mental health practitioners prospering in the era of managed care* (pp. 267–278). Madison, WI: Psychosocial Press.

Hasenfeld, Y. (1974). *Human service organizations.* Ann Arbor: University of Michigan Press.

HMOs cover 73% of workers: Study says plans have cut costs. (1997, January 20). *The Chicago Tribune.*

Hochschild, A. R. (1983). *The managed heart: Commercialization of human feeling.* Berkeley and Los Angeles: University of California Press.

Hoyt, M. (1996). *Constructive therapies.* New York: Guilford.

Leidner, R. (1993). *Fast food, fast talk: Service work and the routinization of everyday life.* Berkeley and Los Angeles: University of California Press.

McIntyre, J. S. (1994). The clinician's view: In R. K. Schreter, S. S. Sharfstein, & C. A. Schreter (Eds.), *Allies and adversaries: The impact of managed care on mental health services* (pp. 163–168). Washington, DC: American Psychiatric Press.

Quinlivan, R., Hough, R., Crowell, A., Beach, C., Hofstetter, R., and Kenworthy, K. (1995). Service utilization and costs of care for severely mentally ill clients in an intensive care management program. *Psychiatric Services, 46*(4), 365–371.

Ritzer, G. (1993). *The McDonaldization of society: An investigation into the changing character of contemporary social life.* Newbury Park, CA: Pine Forge.

Shostak, G. L. (1985). Planning the service encounter. In J. A. Czepiel, M. R. Solomon, & C. F. Surprenant (Eds.), *The service encounter: Managing employee/customer interaction in service businesses* (pp. 243–254). Lexington, MA: Lexington.

Siehl, S., Bowen, D. E., and Pearson, C. M. (1992). Service encounters as rites of integration: An information processing model. *Organizational Science, 3*(4), 537–555.

Skopec, K. A. (1996, December 26). House of cards. *The Chicago Tribune.*

Taylor, F. W. (1947). *The Principles of scientific management.* New York: Harper and Row.

Trabin, T., & Freeman, M. A. (1995). *Managed behavioral healthcare: History, models, strategic challenges and future course.* Tiburon, CA: CentraLink.

Vanstone, M. (1995). Managerialism and the ethics of management. In R. Hugman & D. Smith (Eds.), *Ethical issues in social work* (pp. 120–135). London and New York: Routledge.

Wylie, M. S. (1994). Endangered species. *Networker, 18,* 20–27.

EPILOGUE

Managed care in human services has been described by some people as a tidal surge—catastrophically wiping out everything in its path; some describe it as a sand dune—constantly shifting as it moves forward to claim productive land; others describe it as a phoenix—rising out of the ashes of a devastated system. Rather, managed care in human services is the most recent in a long history of systemic reforms designed to serve the common good with constrained resources.

ISSUES SURROUNDING MANAGED CARE IN HUMAN SERVICES

Four issues emerge from the advent of managed care in the human services. First, there is the human side of managed care. It is care for vulnerable citizens who are marginalized and depend on the largesse of the community, people caught in the tension between cost reduction and quality services. In mental health services, it is the severely and profoundly mentally ill. In child welfare, it is abused and neglected children. These problems, however, are complex, long-standing, and rarely amenable to quick, short-term interventions.

Unfortunately, quality of services continues to receive short shrift. If cost reductions result in improved targeting of resources to better serve these vulnerable citizens, then managed care may have a positive impact. If cost reductions result in elimination of essential services, then once again these vulnerable citizens will bear the brunt of the rationing of limited resources. Rycraft and Mordock, in chapters 2 and 3, describe this tension as the hallmark of managed care in child welfare. Hudson documents the failure of the Massachusetts experiment to serve the needs of the severely and profoundly mentally ill, in chapter 4. The DuPage County case, in chapter 9, demonstrates one organization's attempt to meet this challenge. And the Canadian case, in chapter 5, shows how one community worked to build consensus and comprehensive services to serve and protect its neediest citizens.

The second issue emerging from managed care in human services is the threat to survival of existing community service networks. For the most part, organizations in these networks operate within annual budgets of less than $500,000. Originally established by volunteers to address local problems, over time these community-based, volunteer-run organizations patched together their resources to transform themselves into volunteer-supervised integrated service systems. Building community consensus is a slow and often painstaking process. In chapter 5 Thomlison et al. provide an example of how to refashion the continuum of care, retain community support, and sustain the long-term commitment required to bring about success.

The third issue arising from managed care in human services is the value placed on a rational, logical, reductionist system for meeting human service needs. Such a system is characterized by a closed loop of decision processes, predicated on standardized best practices. It requires a capacity to collect, manage, and apply a vast quantity of information to achieve measurable outcomes. It also assumes that professional services are interchangeable and that substitutability is a desirable and achievable goal.

As several authors have pointed out, these assumptions start from a dubious premise. Our knowledge about the relationship among intervention, outcome, and substitutability is rudimentary. Few resources and little time or money have been spent on studying these issues. Rycraft and Mordock maintain that until understanding these issues becomes vitally important to purchasers of services, little headway is likely to be made in improving this situation.

The fourth issue concerns the structure of managed care in human services. Many state social service and health plans carve out long-term behavioral health care for individuals with chronic conditions. Hudson demonstrates the negative effects of a carved-out system. The DuPage case, however, depicts a positive response to the implementation of a carved-out system designed to serve individuals with continuing and chronic needs.

HOW ARE HUMAN SERVICE ORGANIZATIONS RESPONDING TO MANAGED CARE INITIATIVES?

This question dominates discussion at virtually every gathering of human service professionals. The variety of organizational responses can be attributed to the fact that appropriate strategies fall along a continuum. At one extreme are organizations that choose to disregard managed care in whole or in part. This niche-type response is possible because alternative funding sources exist (for example, United Way), states carve out services, or the relatively small volume of business generates insignificant revenue for the organization (for example, counseling services).

In responding to managed care, a human service organization can choose to find and fill a niche. Here the organization becomes the sole or largest provider of a particular service for a particular population or problem. Thus the organization is less vulnerable to external forces. This strategy was evident with the innovators at Provident Counseling, described in chapter 6. However, as that case demonstrates, the organization's viability can be threatened. In the DuPage case, the mental health organization focused on serving the severely and profoundly ill.

Progressing along the continuum, an organization can choose to expand. Not unlike the niche strategy, the human service organization seeks to provide a broader range of services. New services are usually related to the core mission of the organization, so there is less adaptation of and disruption to operations. An example is DePelchin Children's Center, in chapter 8, which developed a complete, comprehensive continuum of care for children. However, expansion is likely to push the human service organization into the marketplace with large medical centers and hospital networks that are formidable competitors.

A human service organization can choose to pursue a collaborative strategy in order to retain some organizational autonomy. The continuum of care is developed across a group of organizations. Unlike the expansion strategy in which a single organization provides the service array, an integrated network pools services into an array. Each organization retains its autonomy while cost sharing and cooperating on delivery of services under a managed care contract. In some instances, administrative functions may also be pooled. Thomlison et al. describe one such effort.

Another kind of collaboration involves pooling resources to create new organizational forms such as joint ventures, mergers, or acquisitions. Sidwell's description of TexCare, in chapter 3, is a prime example of this approach to collaboration. Mergers and acquisitions are becoming more common in human services. Mergers among nonprofit organizations or, more uncommonly, between nonprofit and for-profit organizations are becoming the leading edge of development in this area.

WHAT WORKS?

The only common denominator evident among these cases is that there is no one-size-fits-all solution. A combination of organizational and environmental factors will determine locally appropriate, acceptable, and ultimately successful responses to the challenges imposed by managed care in human services. Administrators and the human service organizations they lead must be flexible, thoughtful, and attuned to the forces at work in their environments. They must discern threats and opportunities and be sensitive to tensions within the organization. Each organization's strengths and weaknesses will influence its responses to managed care initiatives in its community. Administrators must know at what level and in which arena the organization can operate in order to survive in such a dynamic environment. In the future, more administrators of human service organizations may also have to consider joining with others to create a new organization rather than attempt to survive alone in the marketplace.

For the human service organization that chooses to work within the managed care environment, and for its leadership, there are two additional caveats. First, the organizational transformation must be appropriately anchored to the culture of the human service entity. Not all organizations are well suited for managed care. The Provident Counseling and DuPage County cases demonstrate the challenges and problems that face transforming organizations.

The second caveat concerns time. Creating and institutionalizing change takes a long time. Managed care requires a fundamental change in the design and delivery of human services. It requires a fundamental change in how business is conducted in a market-oriented environment. All four cases in part 2 of this volume illustrate these challenges to the customary way of providing human services.

WHAT DOESN'T WORK?

The status quo does not work. In chapter 10, Crotty delineates a fundamental challenge to the helping relationship permeating the operational environment of managed care. He convinces us that our emphasis must be on helping those with chronic problems become fully functioning members of society.

Organizations cannot ignore the realities of this new operational environment. Administrators must have contingency plans and strategies for initiating change. To ignore the environment is to doom the organization. Another operational reality is information management. Administrators of human service organizations must become more knowledgeable about and comfortable with the use of information. Service data and financial data are necessary components of a managed care system. If administrators cannot utilize data effectively, they will be at the mercy of administrative service organizations and contracting agents. Mordock and Rycraft articulate clearly and succinctly the importance of data management for human services under managed care.

Finally, under managed care, low bidding to obtain contracts is no longer viable. In the past, human service organizations would underbid or low-bid their services in order to secure state contracts. They would then supplement income from state contracts with funding from other revenue sources. In today's risk-sharing, cost-containing environment, low bidding on contracts will place the human service organization at risk of bankruptcy or worse, business closure. Only a large organization might be able to continue this practice, but even then at considerable risk to its solvency. Risk sharing is a more dangerous practice than in the past. In today's resource-constrained environment, assuming inordinate risk can be the death knell of the human service organization.

INDEX

227